Advance Praise for *The Finding Solid Ground Program Workbook*

"*Finding Solid Ground* is easily one of the most helpful books available on the treatment of clinical dissociation. Based on an extended clinical research study, this guide is highly recommended for those who seek concrete, evidence-based guidance in this area. Equally recommended is the associated workbook, which provides detailed and compassionate information and exercises for clients struggling with dissociative challenges."

—**John Briere**, Ph.D., the professor emeritus of psychiatry, Keck School of Medicine, University of Southern California, author, *Treating Risky and Compulsive Behavior in Trauma Survivors*

"*Finding Solid Ground* is an enormous contribution to the field of trauma: the first book on trauma and dissociation written by authors who are both scholars and clinicians. They build a solid ground of research evidence to support an understanding of dissociation combined with practical applications that can be easily integrated into psychotherapy or serve as a stand-alone treatment. Well done!"

—**Janina Fisher**, Ph.D., author of *Healing the Fragmented Selves of Trauma Survivors, Transforming the Living Legacy of Trauma,* and *The Living Legacy Flip Chart*

"*Finding Solid Ground* provides invaluable resources on the treatment of dissociative trauma-related disorders. The authors are educators *par excellence* who have used their expertise as researchers and clinicians to produce a highly readable overview of dissociation along with treatment guidelines and exercises. Their innovative TOP DD studies offer empirical support for their approach. A major contribution!"

—**Christine A. Courtois**, Ph.D., ABPP, licensed psychologist, consultant/trainer, author, co-editor, *The Treatment of Complex Traumatic Stress Disorders* (2020)

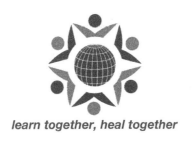

learn together, heal together

The Finding Solid Ground Program Workbook

OVERCOMING OBSTACLES IN TRAUMA RECOVERY

Hugo J. Schielke, Bethany L. Brand,
and Ruth A. Lanius

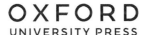

OXFORD
UNIVERSITY PRESS

OXFORD
UNIVERSITY PRESS

Oxford University Press is a department of the University of Oxford. It furthers
the University's objective of excellence in research, scholarship, and education
by publishing worldwide. Oxford is a registered trade mark of Oxford University
Press in the UK and certain other countries.

Published in the United States of America by Oxford University Press
198 Madison Avenue, New York, NY 10016, United States of America.

Library of Congress Cataloging-in-Publication Data
Names: Schielke, Hugo J., author. | Brand, Bethany L., author. |
Lanius, Ruth A., author.
Title: The finding solid ground program workbook : overcoming obstacles in trauma recovery /
Hugo J. Schielke, Bethany L. Brand, Ruth A. Lanius.
Description: New York, NY : Oxford University Press, 2022. |
Includes bibliographical references and index.
Identifiers: LCCN 2022010876 (print) | LCCN 2022010877 (ebook) |
ISBN 9780197629031 (paperback) | ISBN 9780197629055 (epub) |
ISBN 9780197629062
Subjects: LCSH: Post-traumatic stress disorder—Treatment. |
Dissociative disorders—Treatment. | Psychotherapy—Methodology.
Classification: LCC RC552.P67 S325 2022 (print) | LCC RC552.P67 (ebook) |
DDC 616.85/21—dc23/eng/20220510
LC record available at https://lccn.loc.gov/2022010876
LC ebook record available at https://lccn.loc.gov/2022010877

DOI: 10.1093/med-psych/9780197629031.001.0001

Printed in Canada by Marquis Book Printing

CONTENTS

PREFACE

ABOUT THE FINDING SOLID GROUND PROGRAM

The challenges that trauma survivors often face can feel overwhelming. Trauma can cause or contribute to many problems for survivors, including:

- feeling "too much" (feeling strong or overwhelming feelings or urges)
- feeling "too little" (not feeling emotions or body sensations) or feeling numb
- feeling disconnected from their bodies
- feeling disconnected from other people
- feeling confused or having difficulty thinking clearly
- losing track of time, sense of place (where they are), or what is happening
- having difficulty noticing when things are safer
- having trauma-related emotions, memories, and physical sensations from the past intrude into the present
- having difficulty maintaining healthy self-care and relationships, and
- suffering from a variety of medical problems and illnesses, many of which may be exacerbated by stress.

Despite wanting to heal and feel safer, trauma survivors may not believe that healing or getting and feeling safer is possible. Many may unfairly believe they do not deserve to feel better. People who have experienced trauma may also do risky or unhealthy things in an effort to get some relief—even if only for a short time—from their emotional pain and symptoms. (Unfortunately, although it may not be readily apparent to trauma survivors, these risky and unhealthy behaviors contribute to keeping them feeling unsafe, which keeps them from making better progress toward healing and recovery.)

Learning new ways of doing things is hard for all of us—especially if someone feels confused and conflicted about getting safer and doing things differently, as people who have experienced trauma often do. It often does not feel OK to make changes that go against "lessons" or "rules" learned as part of being hurt or mistreated. (For example, people who have experienced trauma may believe they do not deserve to feel good, or safe, or happy, even though these thoughts are not true or fair—people who have experienced trauma *do* deserve to feel good, safe, and happy.) Furthermore, talking about trauma-related reactions can sometimes remind people of past trauma and lead to trauma-related reactions. This in turn may increase the person's urges to engage in unhealthy, risky, and unsafe behaviors.

Finally, each of the experiences described above can interfere with attention, concentration, and memory, making it difficult to take in, remember, and use new information. These problems can make it difficult to learn and remember new healthy coping skills that are necessary to heal from the impact of trauma.

These are the challenges faced by trauma survivors.

When trauma happens repeatedly in relationships that were supposed to be safe and loving, when it occurs in childhood, and/or when it happens in relationships with caregivers, it is referred to as *complex trauma*. Individuals who have experienced complex trauma are likely to have particular difficulty with feeling too much or too little and are at greater risk for using unhealthy, unsafe, or risky ways of managing their feelings and symptoms.

In order to help people who have experienced trauma, and the therapists who strive to help them recover, we developed this program, which we call the *Finding Solid Ground* program. This workbook can serve as a guide to managing and reducing trauma-related symptoms and reactions for people who have been traumatized. Therapists are likely to find the program's materials useful in their work with people who have experienced trauma. (We use the terms "people who have experienced trauma"/"been traumatized," "trauma survivors," and "individuals with trauma histories" interchangeably throughout this workbook.)

ABOUT THIS WORKBOOK

This workbook contains the Information Sheets and exercises that are the foundation for the Finding Solid Ground program. (We'll talk more about these in the "Overview of the Finding Solid Ground Program Materials" section below.) We have also created a companion book called *Finding Solid Ground: Overcoming Obstacles in Trauma Treatment*. This companion book provides the theoretical and clinical rationale for the Finding Solid Ground program, reviews research relevant to the Finding Solid Ground program, and offers guidance to therapists working with people who have experienced trauma. Although developed primarily as a book for therapists, trauma survivors and their loved ones interested in understanding the foundations of this program and trauma's impact may find the companion book informative, too.

In our attempt to make this workbook user-friendly, we do not review the theory and underlying research supporting the educational materials in the Finding Solid Ground program in detail, but we do provide a *very* brief overview of it here to help readers know that this approach is grounded in research and the clinical literature.

BRIEF OVERVIEW OF THEORY AND RESEARCH

For trauma survivors, it can sometimes feel like an unending cycle of symptoms and suffering. The process of healing trauma-related symptoms, patterns of behavior, and long-held but unfair trauma-related beliefs can be daunting. But as the research reviewed in the companion book illustrates, people who have experienced trauma, including complex trauma, *can* make meaningful and important progress in treatment. You *can* learn how to heal, recover, and grow—and this program can help you do it.

As trauma therapists who are also researchers, we developed this program based on the clinical literature and research. Trauma experts and research support an approach that emphasizes helping people recognize and understand trauma-related symptoms and how to get and feel safer, learn healthy and safe ways to manage trauma-related symptoms (including feeling too much or too little), and develop healthy coping and relationships (including, and especially, with themselves). This educational, stabilizing approach needs to be emphasized throughout treatment and is especially important in the beginning of treatment for complex trauma. The educational approach offered in the Finding Solid Ground program is consistent with the treatment approach advocated by complex trauma experts (see the Resources section at the end of this workbook for treatment guidelines and books related to complex trauma).

We have also been active in researching the assessment and treatment of trauma-related problems and disorders. We are part of a group of researchers who collaborated on the Treatment of Patients with Dissociative Disorders (TOP DD) studies. The TOP DD research team[1] is made up of experts who help people with trauma histories, and the TOP DD studies contributed to the development of the Finding Solid Ground program. The TOP DD studies and studies conducted by other researchers around the world have consistently shown that people who have experienced trauma can benefit from trauma treatment. As part of the TOP DD Network study, we offered the first version of this program to individuals who have experienced trauma and their therapists. The results of the TOP DD Network study indicated that survivors of trauma made meaningful improvements in reducing and managing trauma-related symptoms and emotions. In addition to learning healthy ways to get their needs met safely, survivors in the TOP DD Network study also reduced their use of risky and unhealthy behaviors.

---

[1] The TOP DD collaborators: Bethany L. Brand, Hugo J. Schielke, Frank W. Putnam, Richard J. Loewenstein, Amie Myrick, Karen Putnam, Ellen K. K. Jepsen, Willemien Langeland, Kathy Steele, Catherine Classen, Suzette Boon, Paul A. Frewen, and Ruth A. Lanius.

However, we have some important disclaimers to share:

1. Although participants showed meaningful improvements and said that these improvements were due to participating in the program, only studies that use random assignment of participants to a "control group" and to a "treatment group" can prove convincingly that the program caused the changes. The TOP DD Network study did not have a control group— only a treatment group where everyone participated in the program—so we cannot be certain that the psychoeducational program caused the improvements. (We are currently in the process of preparing a randomized controlled study.)

2. All of the trauma survivors who worked on this program as part of the TOP DD Network study were in treatment with a therapist who had at least some training in treating trauma. Therapists and survivors worked through the first version of the Finding Solid Ground program together, which also involved watching educational videos that described the information we present in this book's information sheets and written and practice exercises. (The videos are part of ongoing research trials and are not available to the public as of the writing of this book.) That means each therapist planned and provided each client's treatment, and the program was an *addition* to therapy. We have not yet conducted a study to determine how individuals who have experienced trauma and who are not in individual therapy respond to this educational program without the assistance of a therapist or without watching the videos.

We want to be clear: The Finding Solid Ground program is a research-informed *educational* program that has been researched and will continue to be studied. It is *not* treatment. We recommend that readers who have experienced trauma consider seeking therapy with a person trained in treating trauma, especially if the survivor is struggling with safety problems including unsafe relationships or serious unhealthy behaviors or symptoms that interfere with their quality of life. Readers need to make their own decisions about whether to do this program and, if they decide to try all or parts of the educational program, whether to do it alone or to work on the program with the assistance of a therapist.

To support those working with treatment providers, we make suggestions about "talking to your therapist" or "talking to a treatment provider" about various topics in this workbook. If you are not working with a therapist, please consider these prompts as invitations to consider whether it might be helpful to begin working with a therapist. We especially encourage you to consider finding and working with a therapist if you are struggling with symptoms and feelings that make it difficult for you to function day to day, cause you to feel hopeless, or seriously interfere with living well. There is a list of resources at the back of this workbook that might assist you in finding a therapist in your area who has been trained in helping trauma survivors heal, as well as a list of resources that may be helpful if you need help urgently.

Whether alone or with a therapist, we advise against trying to rush through the materials. Instead, we recommend going through them at a pace that feels manageable to you. The goal is to learn and practice new ways of helping yourself manage and heal the impacts of trauma. Reaching this goal will require repeated practice of what you will be learning over time. (We offer more detailed recommendations about this in "Welcome to the Finding Solid Ground Program: An Introduction to the Program and How to Get the Most Out of It," which follows this preface.)

THE FINDING SOLID GROUND PROGRAM'S EDUCATIONAL TARGETS, RESEARCH, AND CLINICAL FOUNDATIONS

The Finding Solid Ground program targets symptoms and difficulties that often emerge in the wake of having experienced trauma. As part of this process, the program provides education about healthy, healing- and-recovery-focused ways to manage and reduce trauma-related symptoms, emotions, thoughts, and behaviors—recovery-focused skills that make it possible for trauma survivors to get and feel safer as they put this information and these skills into practice.

There were many sources of knowledge, expertise, and research that guided the development of the Finding Solid Ground program. Those that most directly informed the program are cited as references and listed in the Resources section of this workbook. Clinical theory about complex trauma, trauma treatment research, and expert guidelines and recommendations for treating complex trauma and dissociative disorders guided the program's development. The companion book for therapists reviews and acknowledges these important sources of clinical and research wisdom. We are deeply appreciative of all the experts, researchers, and trauma survivors who have contributed to our current understanding of the many paths and techniques that can contribute to healing from trauma. We especially want to acknowledge the Trauma Disorders Program at Sheppard Pratt, where the first two authors received training in, and provided treatment for, trauma-related disorders. This program, under the direction of Richard J. Loewenstein, MD, has helped many people with trauma histories make meaningful progress toward getting and feeling safer. This program has also trained many mental health care providers (including psychiatrists, psychologists, social workers, and nurses) in how to help people with extensive trauma histories.

The Finding Solid Ground psychoeducational program was the core of the TOP DD Network study. As reviewed in the companion book, the participants in the TOP DD Network study showed a wide range of meaningful improvements while using the program. We have used feedback from the individuals and therapists who participated in the TOP DD Network study to refine the program materials. The TOP DD Network study co-investigator, Dr. Hugo Schielke, has been using this refined program in trauma symptom management treatment groups and has further refined the program based on feedback from these group members.

The TOP DD slogan is "work together, learn together." This is the philosophy that has guided the exchange of ideas that led to the initial development and repeated refinements of the Finding

Solid Ground program. Based on our research and clinical work using this program, we believe that the program presented in this workbook offers useful information toward getting and feeling safer.

OVERVIEW OF THE FINDING SOLID GROUND PROGRAM MATERIALS

The program we share in this workbook provides education through a series of information sheets and written and practice exercises that aim to help trauma survivors in several ways. First, the program is geared to provide information about trauma-related symptoms; early "warning signs" that might indicate that the person is becoming distressed or overwhelmed; and healthy, recovery-focused ways of managing and reducing these symptoms. Second, the program teaches healthy ways of managing and relating to emotions, increasing healthy self-compassion, and reducing unfair trauma-based thoughts. (Trauma-based thoughts can lead to shame and harsh self-criticism, and such thoughts can contribute to feeling too much or too little and urges to engage in risky/unhealthy behaviors.) We also seek to increase trauma survivors' awareness of what can lead or contribute to urges to do things that are risky, unhealthy, or unsafe and to offer help about how to get healthy needs met safely.

The TOP DD Network study and other research shows that individuals who have experienced trauma *can be helped to heal and grow.* We, the authors of this workbook, sincerely hope our program also helps you, our readers, heal from trauma. We hope that it helps you, like our research participants, *find solid ground.*

The Finding Solid Ground program covers 30 topics organized into eight modules, with an information sheet and accompanying written and practice exercises for each topic.

- Each information sheet presents an overview of a particular skill or topic, and each subtopic is presented in its own "focus box."
- There is also a set of written and practice exercises for each of the 30 topics. Written and practice exercise sets offer opportunities to apply the information presented in the corresponding information sheet. We encourage you to work on the materials at your own pace. We expect that most readers will need to work on the materials slowly so that they do not get overwhelmed by feeling too much or too little. In general, each exercise set's practice exercise will follow the written exercises. The exception to this is in the first set of grounding exercises, as we want to encourage people to make sure they are grounded before doing work in this program.

After an introductory welcome that describes the program's goals, content, and recommendations on how to get the most out of the program, you will find a script for grounding, followed by the program's information sheets and exercises. Materials and the sequence in which they are presented are informed by years of discussions among experts in treating and researching traumatized individuals, a panel of trauma survivors who reviewed and critiqued the materials, feedback from participants in the TOP DD Network study, and feedback from people who participated in groups using the program materials. Over the course of the workbook, topics build on the material presented in prior information sheets and work done in prior written and practice exercises. We think it is probably best for most people to start at the beginning and work straight through the workbook materials rather than skipping around.

We encourage patience and healthy self-compassion to trauma survivors, therapists, and group facilitators as they work through the program. We hope that the program enhances readers' self-understanding and compassion, management of trauma-related difficulties, and healing. As Dr. Richard Kluft, a pioneering trauma expert, has noted, "The slower you go, the faster you'll get there."

Now that we have introduced you to the more theoretical and research-based aspects of the program, we are going to shift the focus and tone for the rest of the workbook. We will now directly begin to encourage you to learn all you can about healing from the impact of trauma. Let's get started!

WELCOME TO THE FINDING SOLID GROUND PROGRAM: AN INTRODUCTION TO THE PROGRAM AND HOW TO GET THE MOST OUT OF IT

A NOTE FROM THE PROGRAM'S CREATORS

Welcome to the Finding Solid Ground program! We created this program to help people who have experienced trauma and have trauma-related symptoms (including dissociation) learn how to get and feel safer. This program makes use of everything we have learned from our research and therapy work. From this work, we know that you have a lot of strengths and creativity that have helped you survive and (cautiously) seek help toward healing. We are very glad that you are choosing to take these steps for yourself!

We want you to know that if getting and feeling safer is a difficult topic for you, you are definitely not alone. There are very understandable reasons why getting and feeling safer can be hard for people who have experienced trauma. We'll be talking about these reasons as part of this program. We also want you to know that although getting and feeling safer involves hard work, it is absolutely possible. The information we will be providing throughout this program has helped many people. Based on our research and experience, we believe that it can help you, too.

Over the course of this program, we will work together to help you learn:

- **How what you are going through makes sense given a history of trauma.**
  This information will include helping you understand symptoms related to trauma; trauma's effects on the brain; and common trauma-driven impacts on people's feelings, relationships, and views about themselves and the world.

- **How to help yourself (including your brain) heal from the effects of trauma, starting with healthy ways to manage trauma-related symptoms,** including experiences of feeling too much or too little.
- **How to have healthy relationships—starting with your relationships with yourself, with all of who you are.** For those of you with dissociative self-states or "parts" (aspects of yourself that are very different and separate from other parts of yourself), this will involve learning how to develop better relationships between these different parts of yourself. For those who do not have dissociative self-states, you may find the exercises and suggestions included for people with parts helpful if you approach them thinking about different roles you play in your life, or different aspects of who you are, or different aspects of your experience ("part of me feels this way, another part of me feels differently").

To help you put what you are learning into practice, we provide written and practice exercises for each topic we discuss. Purchasers of this book can reproduce its materials for their own personal clinical use only (either as a patient or as a therapist).

If all of this feels like a lot, that is understandable. We are talking about a healing process that will take time—so we encourage you to be very patient with yourself. Go through this program at a pace that feels manageable to you. As Dr. Richard Kluft, a well-known expert in the trauma field, has said, "The slower you go, the faster you'll get there."

We know you can get there by working this program diligently each week, at a slow pace. To give yourself time to practice what you'll be learning, **we recommend going no faster than one topic per week.** You'll make the best progress by taking time to practice what you're learning in each topic's information sheet and written and practice exercises. Slowly but surely, you'll get there. (And if you are working with a therapist, please talk to them about any difficulties or questions that come up along the way!)

HOW TO GET THE MOST OUT OF THIS PROGRAM

As you go through this process, please be patient and gentle with yourself, remembering that *learning takes time and practice.* It takes time to learn something new, and it takes repeated practice to be able to do new things well. Regular practice helps us learn better and faster.

Please also remember that it is not fair to expect to be able to do new things perfectly (or even well) before you (1) have been taught how to do them, (2) understand how to do them, and (3) have lots of practice doing them.

Why do we encourage you to remember this? Unfortunately, people who have experienced trauma often find it difficult to be fair with themselves. (We will be talking about the reasons for this as part of this program, too.) If this is true for you, it could mean that you might unfairly expect yourself to remember something very new and/or different the first time you hear it. Or you might unfairly expect yourself to be able to do something perfectly, right away, once you have been taught how to do it—or maybe even *before* you've been taught how to do it. But these expectations are not fair: The reality is that learning how to do new things well takes time and practice for *everyone*.

It may help to think of an example: Consider learning a language or a musical instrument very different than any you have spoken or played before. Not only are you learning a lot of new information, but you are also learning how to do something very different than what you have done before. It would not be fair to expect someone else to learn to speak a new language or play a new instrument without a lot of practice, would it? If that's true for others, then it is only fair that it is also true for you.

We all do better when we acknowledge that doing new things is often hard at first and that it gets easier (and we get better) as we practice doing them. This is why we encourage you to regularly practice what you are learning. We hope you will set aside time each day to practice the skills you will be learning. *We especially recommend practicing skills at times you do not urgently need them.* Repeatedly practicing new skills when you do not actively need them will make it much easier to use them when you are feeling too much or too little. (Put another way, practicing skills when you aren't feeling too much or too little prepares you to use them successfully when you are!)

As you learn, it is also important to make sure that you are noticing and giving yourself credit for the work you are doing to help yourself even if you cannot (or cannot always) do everything you are learning just yet. ("Yet" being the most important word of that sentence—with practice, you will get there!) Even though the path to healing is sometimes very difficult and can take tremendous work, you can help yourself work toward healing and building a life you actually feel good about.

As you go through this process, from time to time you might doubt yourself, or this program's ability to help you, or your ability to heal. That is understandable. Remember to take it an hour or a day at a time, knowing the goal is your recovery. We will help you take it day by day, minute by minute, or second by second, whatever you need. Please feel free to reread this if you need to borrow some hope from us!

If you feel like you are losing hope, please talk about this with your therapist or a treatment provider or counselor who can help carry hope for you and lend you some of theirs.

We know that if you stick with the process, you can heal and build a life that makes sense and matters to you. You have a lot of strengths within you. If it does not feel like you do, know that this program will help you find them!

Sticking with this work is the most important part. Because making these kinds of changes is difficult, it can be hard to get and stay motivated to do the things that will help you gradually feel better. It takes real effort, every day. If you want to build muscle, you have to use your muscles often; it is the same with developing skills that will give you better control in your life. If you want to get better at managing your symptoms, you have to practice the skills every day.

Many people going through this process sometimes feel a fear of changing how they do things. This is normal and part of what it means to be human. Human beings are often very afraid of change. Whenever this happens, please bring it up with your therapist. You do not need to be ashamed of those feelings. This program can help you work on fear of change and other feelings, as can your therapist.

Do you doubt whether you are worth the time to do this program? Do you doubt whether you are worth making your healing a priority? It is OK if you have doubts. If and when you do, consider rereading this introduction, and remember: Many people who have helped themselves heal from trauma had doubts during the course of their treatment. You can do it! Persistence is the key!

Your healing, starting with getting safer, is a priority. Step by step, you can get there.

AN OVERVIEW OF TOPICS COVERED IN THE PROGRAM

Module (*Goals*)	Topics covered
1. **Grounding** *(Goal: Prevent getting overwhelmed by learning how to help yourself when feeling too much or too little)*	Topic 1: Grounding: When, How, Why
	Topic 2: Signs You Are Starting to Get Ungrounded and Healthy Ways to Get Grounded
	Topic 3: 101 Healthy Ways to Get Grounded
2. **Separating Past from Present** *(Goals: Noticing when the present is safer than past, being aware of current resources, learning how to contain traumatic intrusions)*	Topic 4: Separating Past From Present: When, How, Why
	Topic 5: Using Imagery to Help Separate Past from Present
	Topic 6: Separating Past from Present: Managing 90/10 Reactions
3. **Additional Foundations** *(Goal: Learning additional ways to help yourself make progress toward getting and feeling safer)*	Topic 7: More Healthy Ways to Help Yourself When You're Feeling Too Much
	Topic 8: How to Help Yourself Heal the Impact of Trauma on the Brain
	Topic 9: Managing Crisis-Level Feelings
	Topic 10: The Importance of Self-Compassion in the Healing Process
	Topic 11: Managing Trauma-Based Thoughts
4. **Getting and Feeling Safer, Part 1** *(Goal: Learning how to recognize and interrupt patterns that can contribute to risky, unhealthy, or unsafe behavior or get in the way of getting and feeling safer)*	Topic 12: Recognizing and Planning How to Manage Challenging Situations
	Topic 13: Getting Healthy Needs Met Safely
	Topic 14: Why People Who Have Experienced Trauma Sometimes Do Risky, Unhealthy, or Unsafe Things, and How to Get Healthier and Safer
	Topic 15: The Cycle of Unhealthy Behavior and How to Break Out of It
	Topic 16: Understanding and Reducing Trauma-Related Reactions

Module (*Goals*)	Topics covered
5. **Addressing Trauma-Based Thinking** *(Goal: Learning how to identify and reduce trauma-based thinking)*	Topic 17: Shifting from Trauma-Based Thoughts to Healing-Focused Thinking
	Topic 18: Making the Decision to Get Healthier and Safer
6. **Getting and Feeling Safer, Part 2** *(Goal: Learning more ways to help yourself recognize, interrupt, and reduce patterns that can contribute to risky, unhealthy, or unsafe behavior)*	Topic 19: Working to Calm Your Alarm System
	Topic 20: Feeling Too Much or Too Little and Your Window of Tolerance
	Topic 21: Helping Yourself Recognize Signs That Your Risk of Doing Unhealthy or Unsafe Things Is Increasing
7. **Improving Your Relationship with Emotions, Body Sensations, and Aspects of Self** *(Goal: Learning how to improve your relationship with all aspects of who you are)*	Topic 22: How to Help Your Feelings Help You
	Topic 23: Why Naming Feelings Can Be Difficult
	Topic 24: Naming Feelings
	Topic 25: Self-Understanding Through Compassion: Accepting All Your Feelings
	Topic 26: Safely Practicing Noticing and Naming Feelings
	Topic 27: Guilt, Shame, and Self-Compassion
8. **Sticking With the Process and Building on Progress** *(Goal: Learning how to keep building on the progress you've been making)*	Topic 28: Feeling Safe Takes LOTS of Practice
	Topic 29: Let the Good Times Roll—Learning How to Allow Good Feelings and Positive Experiences
	Topic 30: You Have Learned a Lot—How You Can Keep Healing

Grounding

Grounding offers powerful help toward managing and reducing symptoms related to trauma.

This module will help you learn:

- what grounding is
- how to help yourself get grounded
- signs you are getting ungrounded.

This module will help you practice:

- getting grounded
- noticing signs you are getting ungrounded
- getting grounded when you first begin to notice getting ungrounded.

This work will help you learn how to prevent yourself from getting overwhelmed by learning healthy, healing-focused ways to help yourself when you start to feel too much or too little.

GROUNDING SCRIPT

Grounding is a recovery-focused skill that offers powerful help toward managing and reducing symptoms related to trauma, including feeling too much or too little.

There are two core grounding skills: *orienting yourself to the present* and *anchoring yourself in the present*. Let's try them now.

Grounding, Step 1: Orienting yourself to the present

Orienting yourself to the present involves using your mind to help yourself connect to the here and now.

Think to yourself: "What year, month, day, and time is it?" "How old am I?" "Where am I?" and "What's the situation?" (Orienting yourself is especially good at helping you connect with the "now" part of the here and now.)

Grounding, Step 2: Anchoring yourself in the present

Once you've oriented yourself to the present, use your five senses to help yourself actively notice and connect to your surroundings in the here and now. (This is referred to as *anchoring yourself in the present*, which is especially good at helping you further connect to the "here" part of the here and now.)

Try doing this now. Look around, describing to yourself what you see. For example: What are the colors of the objects you see? What materials are the objects you see made of? How close or far away are objects from one another? Try describing what you see to yourself in enough detail that if you wrote them down, someone else could imagine them.

What are you hearing? Describe in detail the mixture of different sounds in the environment. Are they high-pitched? Low-pitched? Quiet? Loud? Try describing the sounds to yourself in a way that if you wrote them down, someone else could imagine them.

What smells can you notice? Describe these in detail. (Are they subtle? Strong? Sweet? Spicy?)

What tastes can you notice? If you are drinking or eating something as you do this, notice and describe the colors, flavors, textures, and temperatures of your food or drink to yourself. If your food or drink makes a sound, like crunching (when chewing food) or fizzing (when drinking a soda), describe that to yourself, too.

How about the surfaces around you—what do they feel like? Describe their textures to yourself: Are they rough? Smooth? Are they cool or warm to the touch? Try intentionally choosing different kinds of surfaces to touch and comparing how they feel while describing them to yourself.

When you are finished

Once you are finished, take a moment to notice how you feel now compared to how you felt before you started grounding yourself.

You may notice feeling at least a little more connected to (grounded in) the present. You may also notice feeling a little calmer, more "solid," less confused or scared, and more able to notice and think about what's happening.

Different senses work differently well for anchoring at different times. For example, many people find that the sense of touch and noticing and describing different textures and temperatures helps them get grounded fastest when they most need it. Others like to always start with a deep breath in through their nose (smelling the air) to make sure they are breathing while grounding. (Forgetting to breathe is common among people with trauma histories, and can lead your brain to think that something bad is happening even if it isn't.) To find out what works best for you, try experimenting with the order you describe your senses to yourself in different situations.

Like doing anything new, grounding can be difficult at first, so be sure to give yourself credit for each time you practice and to notice the improvements as they happen. And keep practicing—the more often you take the time to practice orienting to and anchoring in the present, the easier it will get and the more it will help. Also, practicing when you are not overwhelmed will make it much easier to help yourself ground faster when you really need it!

To help yourself get more grounded, please:

- Practice using grounding skills when you do not need them so that you are more ready and able to use them when you need them most.
- Use grounding skills before doing work related to this program (and before therapy, if you are in therapy). This will help you get the most out of the hard work you are doing to help yourself heal, which we are so glad you are doing!
- Begin practicing using grounding skills as soon as you are aware that you may be starting to get overwhelmed or ungrounded (that is, when you start to feel too much or too little, feel disconnected or numb, start to space out, or start to confuse the "here and now" with the "there and then")—including if this happens when working on this program or in therapy.

Each time you help yourself get grounded instead of letting yourself get overwhelmed, you are making meaningful progress toward helping yourself heal. Remember to give yourself credit for this!

GROUNDING: WHEN, HOW, WHY

Information Sheet for Topic 1

When use grounding?

When you first begin to notice . . .

- Feeling "too much" (strong or overwhelming feelings or urges)
- Feeling "too little"
- Feeling disconnected or numb
- Feeling confused or having a hard time thinking clearly
- Losing track of time or where you are
- Having a hard time noticing when things are safer
- Feeling like the past is happening again

How do I help myself get grounded?

1. Start with **orienting yourself to the present**.
   Think to yourself: "What is the current year?" "Month?" "Day?" "Where am I?" "How old am I?"
2. Then work hard to **anchor yourself in the present** by using your five senses to connect to the here and now.

   For example: Describe to yourself at least three things you can see, touch, hear, smell, or taste in great detail (see written exercise).

And keep practicing: The more often you take the time to practice grounding, the easier it will get, and the more it will help!

TIP: Practicing when you are not overwhelmed will make it much easier to help yourself ground faster when you really need it!

Why use grounding?

Grounding helps if you are feeling too much or too little. It helps you feel calmer, "solid," less confused, and more able to notice and think about what is happening in the here and now.

Being grounded keeps you safer:

- Being grounded helps you think clearly.
- Being grounded increases your awareness of what is actually happening.
- Being grounded increases your awareness of the options, choices, and resources available to you.
- Being grounded makes it less likely that you have accidents.
- Being grounded makes it less likely that you make decisions that you regret later.
- Being grounded makes it more likely that you make decisions that will keep you safe and are appropriate for the situation.

Being ungrounded can lead to difficult symptoms and situations:

- Being ungrounded can lead to confusion between the past and the present, feeling too much or too little, and other trauma symptoms.
- Being ungrounded makes it more likely that you make decisions that you regret later.

Being grounded helps you heal:

- Being grounded makes it possible to learn new skills to help yourself (and to notice what helps and what works!).
- Being grounded makes it possible to learn and use healthy ways of relating to yourself and others.
- Being grounded helps you notice when the present is safer than the past, which helps your brain and body heal. (If unsafe things are happening, please let a treatment provider know!)
- Being grounded makes it possible to notice when situations and people are actually OK, and to connect with OK people if you choose to.

EXERCISES FOR TOPIC 1: GROUNDING: WHEN, HOW, WHY

Grounding is a healing-focused skill that offers powerful help toward managing and reducing many symptoms related to trauma, including feeling too much or too little.

People with trauma in their past can sometimes get so worried about something bad happening again that it can be very hard to notice when things are safer in the here and now. People with a history of trauma may also become overwhelmed by emotions, or have very frightening experiences where it feels like the past is happening again—or they may find themselves feeling numb, or disconnected from their emotions, body, or the world around them, or losing track of time in ways that can be very scary.

Grounding can help with each of these trauma-related symptoms. The exercises for this topic will help you practice getting grounded and encourage you to identify your reasons for using grounding skills.

Practice Exercise for Topic 1: Grounding: When, How, Why

To help yourself get more grounded, please:

- Practice using grounding skills when you do not need them so that you are more ready and able to use them when you need them most.
- Use grounding skills before doing work related to this program and before going to therapy. This will help you get the most out of the hard work you are doing to help yourself heal, which we are so glad you are doing!
- Begin using grounding skills as soon as you are aware that you may be starting to get overwhelmed or ungrounded (that is, when you start to feel too much or too little, feel disconnected or numb, start to space out, or start to confuse the "here and now" with the "there and then")—including if this happens when working on this program or in therapy.

> *TIP:* Each time you help yourself get grounded instead of letting yourself get overwhelmed, you are making meaningful progress toward helping yourself heal. Remember to give yourself credit for this!

When grounding (or practicing grounding skills before you need to use them), please practice:

- *Orienting yourself to the present* by reminding yourself of the date, your age, and your situation. (Think to yourself, "What is the current date? Where am I? How old am I?")
- *Anchoring yourself in the present* by using your five senses, describing at least three things you can see, touch, hear, smell, or taste to yourself in great detail.

It can take a while to get good at grounding; practice as often as you can and be patient with yourself—it will get easier! (Many people find it helpful to follow the suggestions of how to do this described in the written exercise on page 8 when they first start.)

Sometimes grounding and working toward getting and feeling safer will be easier than other times. That is OK. Step by step, you will get there!

Three benefits of orienting and anchoring skills:

1. *You do not need any special materials to orient and anchor to the present* (you always have your mind and senses with you!) so . . .

2. You can use these skills to connect to the here and now *whenever you need to help yourself get grounded*, and . . .

3. It is possible to use orienting and anchoring grounding skills without anyone else knowing you are doing it.

This last point is very important to remember if one of your concerns about using grounding skills is that you do not want others to notice you are using a coping skill.

REMEMBER: It is not only OK but also important to notice when you need to take a break from something in order to get grounded. The goal is for you to get and feel safer. Pausing whatever you are doing to help yourself get grounded when you notice that you are feeling too much or too little is actually one of the most powerful ways you can help yourself make progress toward getting and feeling safer.

Written Exercises for Topic 1: Grounding: When, How, Why

Written exercise 1: Practicing orienting and anchoring to the present with writing

The two core grounding skills—orienting to and anchoring yourself in the present—involve describing what you are noticing to yourself in great detail. One good way to practice doing this is to write down what you are trying to help yourself connect to.

Writing things down helps people practice describing things to themselves in detail—especially if they try to write in a way that someone else reading it could picture it in their minds. Writing down what you are noticing can help you connect more deeply with the year, month, day, and time, where you are, your age, and what you are noticing in the here and now with your five senses.

Having said that, different ways of grounding work differently at different times, so if you find that writing gets in the way of you getting and staying grounded, pause and go back to orienting and anchoring yourself to the present without writing.

Willing to give it a try? Bring writing materials to the place that feels most OK to you. (When you first practice something new, it can be helpful to start practicing in situations where the skill is less likely to be necessary.)

Grounding, Step 1: Orienting yourself to the present
Start by *orienting yourself to the present.*
    Write down:

1. The current year, month, day, and time;
2. Your current age; and
3. Where you are.

Then take a moment to look at this.

Grounding, Step 2: Anchoring yourself in the present
Now, work to *anchor yourself in the present.*

1. Look around: What do you see? (What are the colors of the objects you see? What materials are they made of? How close or far away are they from one another?) Write about what you are seeing to yourself in a way that that someone else reading it could picture it in their minds.
2. What are you hearing? Describe the mixture of different sounds in the environment in detail. (Are they high-pitched? Low-pitched? Quiet? Loud? Try describing the sounds in a way that a reader could imagine them.)
3. The surfaces around you—what do they feel like? (Describe their textures: Are they rough? Smooth? Are they cool or warm to the touch?)
4. What smells can you notice? Describe these in detail. (Are they subtle? Strong? Sweet? Spicy?) If you are drinking or eating something as you do this exercise, describe the flavors, textures, and temperatures as well as what it looks like. If it makes a sound (like crunching when you chew it or fizzing like a soda), describe that, too.

Noticing the differences after helping yourself get more grounded
Now take a moment to notice and write down how you feel now compared to how you felt before you started grounding yourself.
    You may notice feeling at least a little more connected to (grounded in) the present. You may also notice feeling calmer, more "solid," less confused or scared, and more able to notice and think about what is happening.
    Practicing grounding when you are not overwhelmed helps create the brain pathways that will help you get grounded faster!

Written exercise 2: Thoughts and feelings related to using grounding skills

Although working to get and stay grounded is a crucial part of helping yourself get and feel safer, you may have mixed feelings about doing something new or different. This week, after practicing grounding by orienting yourself to the present and anchoring yourself in the present, we encourage you to identify *your* reasons for getting grounded and connected with the here and now. We also encourage you to write about any fears you might have about this.[1]

This will help you be aware of *your* pros and cons related to grounding. Being aware of mixed thoughts and feelings can also help you understand and address things that make it difficult to get and stay connected to the here and now.

To help you identify your reasons for using grounding, follow the prompts below to write down your thoughts and feelings about being ungrounded or dissociated (unconnected to the here and now/spaced out/numbed out).

(Note: Some people begin to get ungrounded when they think about being ungrounded. If this happens to you, you will need to work extra hard to keep grounded while you do these exercises.)

1. **Things that make me want to <u>not</u> use grounding skills** (cons of using grounding skills)
   (a) Can you think of any things that might lead you to *not* want to (or not feel like) use grounding skills?

   _____

   _____

   _____

   (b) Are there things that you fear about being grounded/connected to the here and now? If so, please list those here.

   _____

   _____

   _____

   (c) Are there things that you like about being disconnected from the here and now (dissociating)? If so, please list those here.

   _____

   _____

   _____

---

[1] Exercise adapted from Sheppard Pratt Trauma Disorders Program Patient Handouts, v. 2013.

2. **Things that make me _want_ to use grounding skills** (pros of using grounding skills)

    (a) Are there things that you find scary or _dislike_ about being ungrounded or dissociated?
         If so, please list those here.

    If you are having difficulty with this question, consider: When you are ungrounded or
    dissociated, are you more or less likely to confuse the here and now with the there and
    then? Lose track of where you are? Get involved in unhealthy or dangerous situations,
    relationships, or behavior? Have flashbacks?

    _____

    _____

    _____

    (b) Next, we invite you to list _your_ reasons for using grounding skills.

    First, review the reasons for being grounded we discussed in "Why Use Grounding?"
    (see p. 5); circle the ones that are important to you and list them below. Then add any
    other reasons being grounded is important to you.

    Reasons I think it is important to be grounded:

    _____

    _____

    _____

    _____

    _____

3. **Pros and cons of using grounding skills**

    Now let's pull this all together and look at your pros and cons of being grounded. Consider
    the answers you gave to the questions above and list _your_ reasons for using or not using
    grounding skills in the table that follows.

CONS of using grounding skills *(my reasons to NOT use grounding skills)*	PROS of using grounding skills *(my reasons TO use grounding skills)*

We hope this exercise helped you be more aware of your pros and cons of grounding. Grounding plays a big role in getting and feeling safer. Please consider sharing your answers with your individual therapist or a treatment provider—and please talk with them about any questions or concerns you have!

Reference for Topic 1

Trauma Disorders Program, Sheppard Pratt Health System—Patient handouts, v. 2013.

SIGNS YOU ARE STARTING TO GET UNGROUNDED AND HEALTHY WAYS TO GET GROUNDED

Information Sheet for Topic 2

Signs you are starting to get ungrounded or starting to dissociate	Healthy ways to get grounded
Mental signs of getting ungrounded: • Feeling strong anxiety, stress, worry • Feeling overwhelmed • Feeling like it is hard to think clearly or having racing thoughts • Feeling confused, jumbled • Feeling scattered, spacey *Mental signs of dissociation:* • Becoming confused about what is happening (including where you are, who is around, what year it is).	*Mental ways to get grounded:* • Think of the current date, your current age, where you are currently, and notice what is happening around you right now (orienting to the present). • Use your five senses (sight, sound, smell, taste, touch) to connect yourself to and anchor yourself in the here and now (anchoring in the present). (Example: Describe three things around you using a lot of detail.)
Physical signs of getting ungrounded: • Forgetting to breathe • Breathing is quick and shallow. • Feeling intense activity in your body • Feeling tingling, or beginning to feel nothing in your body *Physical signs of dissociation:* • Feeling your body getting numb or feeling tingling sensations • Feeling like you're in a fog, that the world or people around you are far away, or feeling unreal • Feeling like you are disconnecting, fading or spacing out, slipping away • Feeling your body is unreal, feeling unable to move, or feeling your body is changing size • Feeling like you are outside of your body, watching yourself • Seeing with tunnel vision (the edges of what you are looking at get blurry or dark so you can only see what is in the middle of your field of vision)	*Physical ways to get grounded:* • Breathe deeply. • Do active things that feel soothing, like stretching or yoga. • Touch the surfaces around you—what do they feel like? Describe their textures to yourself: Are they rough? Smooth? Are they cool or warm to the touch? Try intentionally choosing different kinds of surfaces to touch, and comparing how they feel while describing them to yourself. • Push your feet into the ground. • Try to tighten all the muscles in your body at the same time for 5 to 10 seconds. • Get unfrozen by beginning to move. If this is difficult, move one finger just a bit, then keep working on getting the movement to be bigger. • Use all your senses to experience the world around you. Explore one object in detail. Example: Look carefully at an orange, feel the texture of its skin, smell it, taste its sweet sharpness, hear yourself chewing it. You can also try this with strong mints, gum, tea or coffee, cold water, ice, and so on. • Use Mindful Walking (preferably without socks and shoes, if this is safe): Walk slowly in a safe place, describing to yourself what you notice.

Why use grounding?

Grounding helps if you are feeling too much or too little. It helps you feel calmer, solid, less confused, and more able to notice and think about what is happening in the here and now.

Being grounded keeps you safer:

- Being grounded helps you think clearly.
- Being grounded increases your awareness of what is actually happening.
- Being grounded increases your awareness of the options, choices, and resources available to you.
- Being grounded makes it less likely that you have accidents.
- Being grounded makes it less likely that you make decisions that you regret later.
- Being grounded makes it more likely that you make decisions that will keep you safe and are appropriate for the situation.

Being ungrounded can lead to difficult symptoms and situations:

- Being ungrounded can lead to confusion between the past and the present, feeling too much or too little, and other trauma symptoms.
- Being ungrounded makes it more likely that you make decisions that you regret later.

Being grounded helps you heal:

- Being grounded makes it possible to learn new skills to help yourself (and to notice what helps and what works!).
- Being grounded makes it possible to learn and use healthy ways of relating to yourself and others.
- Being grounded helps you notice when the present is safer than the past, which helps your brain and body heal. (If unsafe things are happening, please let a treatment provider know!)
- Being grounded makes it possible to notice when situations and people are actually OK, and to connect with OK people if you choose to.

EXERCISES FOR TOPIC 2: SIGNS YOU ARE STARTING TO GET UNGROUNDED AND HEALTHY WAYS TO GET GROUNDED

We hope you have been practicing orienting and anchoring yourself in the present, and that you have started to notice some benefits. We also hope you have been practicing using grounding skills as soon as you start to feel too much or too little.

Please give yourself credit for all the hard work you are doing. Notice little improvements along the way—even if they only happen some of the time! Learning new skills takes time and practice. It is important to notice changes and give yourself credit for doing the hard work involved in learning and practicing new skills. And remember—as you keep practicing, you will be more and more able to help yourself use grounding skills!

We also hope that the Written Exercise for the last topic helped you think through your pros and cons related to grounding, and that you were able to talk about any questions you have with a treatment provider. If you did not do last topic's Written Exercise or have not talked to a treatment provider about any questions you might have, please do—grounding skills are crucially important for your recovery and healing!

Exercises for Topic 2 focus on identifying more ways to help yourself get and stay grounded, starting with **grounding helpers**.

Written Exercises for Topic 2: Signs You Are Starting to Get Ungrounded and Healthy Ways to Get Grounded

Written exercise 1: Identifying grounding helpers
We would like to help you identify **grounding helpers**—things you can carry with you to help yourself get grounded. (Some people refer to this as creating a "grounding kit."[2])

Why? Grounding helpers can help make the two core grounding skills—*orienting* and *anchoring to the present*—easier and more effective.

What kinds of things make for good grounding helpers? Things that are *pleasant to your senses* (that is, touch, sight, smell, sound, taste) and *help you connect to the present*. Possible grounding helpers include:

1. Things that have textures that feel good to you (e.g., a watch or a bracelet with different textures and colors, a smooth stone, clothes or accessories pleasant to touch) (*Senses: sight, touch*)
2. Something small that has a pleasant and strong flavor (e.g., mints) to be able to slowly and mindfully savor the smell and taste of as needed (*sight, sound, touch, taste, smell*)
3. Pictures of places, people, or pets you find calming and soothing (*sight*)
4. Sounds from nature, music, or anything else that you find relaxing or inspiring (*sound*).

---

[2] Sheppard Pratt Trauma Disorders Program, 2013; Vermilyea, 2013.

TIP: It can be very helpful to use things that you KNOW you did not have or that did not exist until after there and then. This will help you KNOW it is not then. The idea is to help yourself orient to the present as quickly and solidly as possible—and having things around that you KNOW are from the near present can be particularly helpful with this!

Take a moment to consider: What items do you already always have with you that you can use as grounding helpers?

_____

_____

_____

_____

_____

What items could you begin to keep with you that you could use as grounding helpers? (Consider adding things related to any of the five senses not included in the objects you already carry with you.)

_____

_____

_____

_____

_____

_____

_____

_____

You have now identified items you can use to help yourself get and stay grounded. Congratulations on identifying grounding helpers!

Written exercise 2: Identifying your signs of getting ungrounded and healthy ways to get grounded

In this exercise, we will help you identify *your* signs that you are getting ungrounded so you can help yourself get grounded as soon as possible. (The earlier you start using grounding skills, the easier it is to help yourself get grounded!) We will also help you identify more healthy ways to help yourself get grounded.

> *TIP:* Remember to pause and focus on getting grounded if you start to get ungrounded! (Helping yourself get and stay grounded is more important than getting through this quickly— and you will actually get through this more quickly if you are grounded!)

Please review the "Signs you are starting to get ungrounded and healthy ways to get grounded" table on page 12.

1. Start by reviewing the column titled "Healthy ways to get grounded."
    As you do:
    - Circle the ways to get grounded that are new to you and you would be willing to try, practice, or do, and
    - Put a checkmark next to any you have tried and found helpful.

2. Then review the column titled "Signs you are starting to get ungrounded or starting to dissociate."
    While reading these, please:
    - Put a mark next to those you have experienced (i.e., identify *your* signs of getting ungrounded), and
    - Think about which of the "healthy ways to get grounded" items you have checked or circled that you could use to help yourself in these situations.
    - In the table below, copy in your signs of getting ungrounded (the signs you marked as having experienced) and the "healthy ways to get grounded" items you identified as helpful to use in these situations.

Signs I am starting to get ungrounded and healthy ways to get grounded

Signs I am starting to get ungrounded or starting to dissociate	Healthy ways to get grounded
Mental signs:	Mental ways to get grounded:
Physical signs:	Physical ways to get grounded:

Practice Exercise for Topic 2: Signs You Are Starting to Get Ungrounded and Healthy Ways to Get Grounded

Congratulations on identifying more ways to help yourself get grounded!

Please take a little time each day to:

- Review the list of "signs you are starting to get ungrounded" and your "signs I am starting to get ungrounded," adding to the list of your signs if you notice more that apply to you. (Keeping these in mind will make it easier to remember to help yourself get grounded as soon and as quickly as possible—the sooner you notice that you are starting to get ungrounded, the easier and quicker it is to get grounded!)
- Review and practice grounding techniques that have helped you or those you are willing to try from your list of "healthy ways to get grounded."
- Work to use grounding skills (including grounding helpers) as soon as you notice signs that you are starting to get ungrounded (feel too much or feel too little/dissociate).

As you work to get and stay grounded:

- *Try to notice which grounding skills work best and when.* Please do not give up or get discouraged if one way of grounding is not working. Keep trying different options from the list of "healthy ways to get grounded" until you find something that works.
- *Please be patient with yourself* as you figure out which safe, healthy ways of getting grounded work for you. *You* are the best person to figure out what you need from minute to minute. If you pay attention to what is happening inside of you, and if you think creatively, you can figure out which healthy way of grounding will work best for you at any moment.

With practice, you can become an expert on grounding yourself. Take one step at a time, and keep up the good work! (And as always, please talk with your therapist or treatment provider about any questions you have.)

> *TIP:* If you are having difficulty staying grounded, **consider checking in with yourself frequently.** Some people check in every half hour, others every 15 minutes or every hour—see what works best for you. Setting reminders on a device can be a big help—as can a grounding check-sheet, like the one on p. 19.[3]

---

[3] Check-sheet adapted from Sheppard Pratt Trauma Disorders Program Patient Handouts, v. 2013.

GROUNDING CHECK-SHEET

This check-sheet can help you notice if (and for how long) you lose track of time. It may also help you notice what was happening that might have made it more difficult to stay grounded.

Please use the "Situation, grounded?" column to briefly describe the situation, adding a checkmark if you are feeling grounded (connected to your body and surroundings). Use the "Grounding skill used" column to note what you did to help ground yourself as needed.

	Situation, grounded?	*Grounding skill used*
7:00 AM		
7:15 AM		
7:30 AM		
7:45 AM		
8:00 AM		
8:15 AM		
8:30 AM		
8:45 AM		
9:00 AM		
9:15 AM		
9:30 AM		
9:45 AM		
10:00 AM		
10:15 AM		
10:30 AM		
10:45 AM		
11:00 AM		
11:15 AM		
11:30 AM		
11:45 AM		
12:00 PM		
12:15 PM		
12:30 PM		
12:45 PM		
1:00 PM		
1:15 PM		
1:30 PM		

	Situation, grounded?	Grounding skill used
1:45 PM		
2:00 PM		
2:15 PM		
2:30 PM		
2:45 PM		
3:00 PM		
3:15 PM		
3:30 PM		
3:45 PM		
4:00 PM		
4:15 PM		
4:30 PM		
5:00 PM		
5:15 PM		
5:30 PM		
5:45 PM		
6:00 PM		
6:15 PM		
6:30 PM		
6:45 PM		
7:00 PM		
7:15 PM		
7:30 PM		
7:45 PM		
8:00 PM		
8:15 PM		
8:30 PM		
8:45 PM		
9:00 PM		
9:15 PM		
9:30 PM		
9:45 PM		
10:00 PM		

	Situation, grounded?	*Grounding skill used*
10:15 PM		
10:30 PM		
10:45 PM		
11:00 PM		
11:30 PM		

References for Topic 2

Trauma Disorders Program, Sheppard Pratt Health System—Patient handouts, v. 2013.

Vermilyea, E. G. (2013). *Growing beyond survival: A self-help toolkit for managing traumatic stress.* Sidran Institute.

101 HEALTHY WAYS TO GET GROUNDED

Information Sheet for Topic 3

Grounding helps you **notice**, **connect with**, and **pay attention to** the **here and now**. The two classic ways of grounding are **orienting yourself to the present** and **anchoring yourself in the present**. We've also talked about **physical ways of getting grounded** and **grounding helpers**.

If you keep the goals of **connecting with** and **paying attention to** the **here and now** in mind, there are lots of healthy, safe things you can do to get and stay grounded. To help you find options that might work well for you, we are sharing a list of "101 Ways to Get Grounded" that people with trauma histories have said work well for them.[4]

Sensory/physical grounding activities

1. Keep your head up (so you can see what is around you), your feet on the ground (do not curl into a ball), and breathe (so your body gets the air it needs to know it is OK).
2. Push your feet into the ground—alternate doing it gently, then pushing hard.
3. Focus on sensations involving your feet—really feel the ground solidly beneath your feet, notice the texture of your socks or shoes against your skin, or if you can, take off your socks and notice how your bare feet feel on the carpet, floor, grass, etc. (Another option: Try rolling a tennis ball with one of your feet without shoes while seated.)
4. Use your senses to connect with the world. (Examples: Notice temperature by holding an ice pack, frozen food, a hot or cold drink, or a heating pad.)
5. Stretch your arms out strong and wide like you are stretching from a good sleep; repeatedly make tight fists, then release the tension.
6. Use muscle relaxation techniques, such as tightening your muscles for 10 seconds and then relaxing them. Pay attention to the different ways your muscles feel before and after you tighten them. Try alternating different muscle groups.

---

[4] The contents of this list are adapted from a list made by people with trauma histories who wanted to share what worked well for them (*The Trauma Disorders Program at Sheppard Pratt Health System, Handouts v.2013*) and feedback from our own patients.

7. Rub or hold a grounding object (a grounding helper) such as a bracelet, watch, necklace, or other jewelry, a stone, a coin, or something that symbolizes recovery, hope, and/or being an adult.

8. Look for colors that you like.

9. Touch your favorite fabric (favorite blanket, shirt, etc.).

10. Smell strong scents that you like, such as peppermint, oranges, scented oils, scented candles, and coffee.

11. Wear your favorite scent or carry a small bottle of it.

12. Have tea, coffee, hot chocolate, or some other favorite nonalcoholic drink. Really notice the taste and temperature.

13. Touch water. Notice the temperature and how it moves.

14. Wash your hands with scented soap.

15. Use a scented lotion.

16. Have a freeze pop or something else that is cold or warm.

17. Get some exercise (even late at night, you can safely do jumping jacks, sit ups, or pushups indoors).

18. Sing along with music you love.

19. Do karaoke.

20. Practice playing an instrument.

21. Jingle your car keys (or something similar).

22. Squeeze a stress ball.

23. Play with a grounding toy (like a squeeze ball or pocket-sized stuffed animal).

24. Play with clay or putty.

25. Play with a Slinky.

26. Wash the dishes. (Focus on the smell of the soap and the feel of the water.)

27. Tidy up your room, bathroom, or car.

28. Clean your home.

29. Take a shower or bubble bath. (Notice the smell of the soap, the feel of the water, the bubbles.)

30. Take care of your hair.

31. Play video games that use motion controls.

32. Play "What's outside my window?" (Look at nature and enjoy and describe in detail what you see.)

33. Garden, paying close attention to the colors, smells, and textures.

34. Go for a walk or hike.

35. Observe and enjoy changes in the season.

36. Ride a bike.

37. Go to the park and swing.

38. Go on a safe adventure. (Examples: Have a picnic, walk in a park, go see a museum exhibit, go to a book store.)
39. Go to a shop with scents, such as a tea shop, coffee shop, candle shop, or cheese shop.
40. Phone a friend.
41. Visit a friend.
42. Play a sport.
43. Bounce a ball.
44. Pet a dog or cat.
45. Hug a pet.
46. Hug or touch a stuffed toy and notice its texture and how it helps you feel safe.
47. Volunteer to help animals or the earth. (Examples: Work at an animal shelter, pick up litter at a park.)
48. Offer to help a friend with a manageable task. (Examples: Help wash each other's cars, take turns cooking or cleaning at each other's homes.)
49. Cook or bake.

Mental grounding activities

1. Orient yourself to your current world: What is your biological age, today's date, your location; who is the current leader of your country; what type of phone, TV, and computer do you use now?
2. Use your five senses to notice the present moment: what the temperature is like, how your clothing feels on your skin, how your feet feel in your shoes.
3. Use "five senses grounding" (describe in detail three things you see, three things you hear, three things you touch, etc.).
4. Practice mindful breathing. (Example: Breathe in for four counts, pause briefly, then breathe out for four counts.)
5. Ask yourself, "Am I grounded?" every 15 minutes. (Set an alarm on your phone or computer to go off every 15 minutes.)
6. Check in with yourself to see how you are feeling (every 15 minutes, if possible).
7. Play "Now Versus Then" (name five things that are better now than in the past).
8. Pay close attention to the experience of eating. (Example: Eat an orange very slowly, noticing its smell, taste, and texture.)
9. Play a card or board game.
10. Play "Counting the Rainbow" (find as many items as you can for each color in the rainbow).

11. Say every other letter of the alphabet or say the alphabet backwards.

12. Count backwards.

13. Play "Current Events." (Examples: How many leaders of different countries can you name, how many capitols of different states or countries can you name?)

14. Name textures. (Touch different surfaces and describe their textures. Example: How does touching a cold water bottle feel compared to touching a towel or a pet?)

15. Observe your surroundings. (Example: What objects do you like in the world around you?)

16. Play "I Spy." (Example: Try to find as many items of your favorite color as you can.)

17. Look for wildlife out your window, or in a yard or park. (Example: How many birds can you see, how many squirrels?)

18. Play "Name That Tune." (Put your music player on shuffle and name the song.)

19. Play trivia games. (Examples: How many actors can you name, how many members of a music group can you name, how many countries in the world can you name?)

20. If you are getting ungrounded while you are a passenger in a car or bus, play car games. (Examples: Look for license plates from various states or countries, look for different models or colors of cars.)

21. Play Sudoku.

22. Do crossword puzzles.

23. Complete a word search.

24. Put a puzzle together.

25. Read a book that helps you feel hopeful or encouraged.

26. Practice learning a new language.

27. Write five positive things about yourself. (If that's too hard, start with two.)

28. Remind yourself that you have lots of strengths! How many can you think of?

Creative grounding activities

1. Do an art or craft project—especially if it is soothing, playful, or funny or makes you feel hopeful.

2. Create a "Five Senses Box" and use it. Put in things you like that use all the senses, such as a soft scarf; mints; a favorite lotion; a music CD that is especially motivating or hopeful; or a picture that helps you feel connected to someone, something, or someplace important to you.

3. Make a collage. (Examples: Use images of beautiful places that are soothing or relaxing, images that represent qualities you are working to develop, images that inspire you or help you feel hope.)

4. Make a scrapbook with pictures of positive experiences or beautiful places.

5. Trace a picture you find beautiful or inspirational and color it in.

6. Make art (draw, color, or paint a picture that has a lot of detail).

7. Engage in a routine that helps you get things done in a way you enjoy. (Example: Fold laundry and really feel the fabric and smell the clean, fresh smell.)

8. Make a grounding bracelet, necklace, or other kind of jewelry—you can touch the beads to help yourself get grounded.

9. Create a mindfulness music playlist; listen to the positive lyrics and the instruments.

10. Paint your fingernails, toenails (if this is something you enjoy).

11. Play energetic, uplifting, inspiring music.

12. Dance.

13. Learn a new dance.

14. Water your plants/garden.

15. Work in the garden or take care of houseplants.

16. Knit or crochet.

17. Sew.

18. Quilt or do needlework.

19. Make pottery.

20. Practice your photography skills.

21. Tie-dye a shirt.

22. Write poetry.

23. Write a story.

24. Write in your journal.

EXERCISES FOR TOPIC 3: 101 HEALTHY WAYS TO GET GROUNDED

We hope you have been practicing orienting and anchoring yourself to the present, and that the exercises from the last topic have helped you notice when you start to get ungrounded. (The sooner you notice that you are starting to get ungrounded, the easier it is to help yourself get grounded again!) We also hope you have been using grounding skills before therapy or before doing any work related to this program.

This topic's exercises focus on helping you identify even more healthy ways to help yourself get and stay grounded.

Written Exercises for Topic 3: 101 Healthy Ways to Get Grounded

Written exercise 1: Identifying more healthy ways to get grounded
As long as you keep the goals of **connecting with** and **paying attention to** the **here and now** in mind, there are lots of healthy, safe things you can do to get and stay grounded. To help you find options that might work well for you, we presented a list of "101 Healthy Ways to Get Grounded" that people with trauma histories have found helpful. Please go through this list. As you do:

- Circle the ways to get grounded that are new to you and you would be willing to try, practice, or do, and
- Put a checkmark next to any you have tried and found helpful.

Written exercise 2: Listing <u>your</u> ways to help yourself get grounded when you start to feel too much or too little
You have been doing a lot of important work in this module! To help you bring all of this work together, please:

- Start by copying the ways to get grounded that you put a checkmark next to (ways that you have tried and found helpful) or circled (ways that are new to you that you are willing to try, practice, or do) from the list of "101 Healthy Ways to Get Grounded" into the list below.
- Then, please go back to page 12 and copy the healthy ways to get grounded that you put a checkmark next to or circled on the "Signs you are starting to get ungrounded and healthy ways to get grounded" table into the list below.
- Finally, you may have other ideas of healthy ways to help yourself get and stay grounded that we did not list in this module. Add those, too! (And feel free to use other paper if you run out of room!) Consider making a copy of this list to carry with you.

Healthy ways to help myself when I feel too much or too little:

_____

_____

_____

_____

_____

_____

_____

_____

_____

_____

_____

_____

_____

_____

_____

_____

_____

_____

_____

Practice Exercise for Topic 3: 101 Healthy Ways to Get Grounded

Congratulations on making a list of healthy things you can do to help yourself when you start to get ungrounded (feel too much or too little)!

Please take a little time each day to:

- Review and practice grounding techniques from your list of "healthy ways to help myself when I feel too much or too little."
- Use grounding skills and do things from this list when you first begin to notice signs that you are starting to feel stressed or overwhelmed, or are beginning to feel too little or dissociate.

You may notice that different grounding techniques have different results at different times—try to notice which techniques work best for which situations.

> *REMEMBER:* Working to help yourself be grounded is a powerful foundation for getting and feeling safer—and can sometimes be very difficult, especially in the beginning. Please be patient and gentle with yourself as you work to get more grounded. Do not give up or get discouraged if one way of grounding is not working. Keep trying different options from your list and this module until you find something that helps, even just a little. Please allow yourself to be creative and flexible when thinking about healthy ways to get and stay grounded.
>
> If you keep practicing and use grounding techniques when you notice signs of feeling too much or too little, you will get better and better at knowing which healthy way of grounding will work best for you at any moment. Talk with your therapist or treatment provider about any questions you have.
>
> Keep up the good work, and make sure to give yourself credit for all the hard work you are doing!

Congratulations on completing the first module!

In the modules that follow, we'll offer additional skills that build on the powerful foundations of orienting yourself to and anchoring yourself in the present. Step by step, you'll get there!

Reference for Topic 3

Trauma Disorders Program, Sheppard Pratt Health System—Patient handouts, v. 2013.

Separating Past from Present

Trying to keep us safer, our minds are on alert for any signs that trauma may be happening again. Unfortunately, because this primes us to notice similarities rather than differences, we can have significant difficulty noticing when situations are safer. In other words, we can have difficulty separating the past from our experience of the present.

This module offers ways to help yourself separate the past from the present. Separating the past from the present helps you see the "here and now" more clearly, which makes it easier to stay grounded and helps you heal.

This module will help you learn:

- what "separating past from present" means
- signs that experiences related to the past might be intruding into the present
- reasons why it can be very difficult to notice how the present is different than the past
- ways to help yourself separate the past from the present.

This module will help you practice:

- noticing and reminding yourself of differences between the past and the present
- catching thinking mistakes that we're all at risk of making—and that can make it difficult to separate the present from the past
- imagery techniques that can help you separate the past from the present
- noticing and managing situations where the past intrudes into the present.

This work will help you notice when the present is safer than the past, be more aware of your current resources and options, and learn how to contain traumatic intrusions.

SEPARATING PAST FROM PRESENT: WHEN, HOW, WHY

Information Sheet for Topic 4

When should I start separating the past from the present?[1]

As soon as you start to feel like . . .

- A situation is "like" or "just like" something from the past, or
- Something from the past is going to happen again.

How do I help myself separate the past from the present?

1. **Start by using your grounding skills** to *orient* and *anchor* yourself to the present.
   It is always easier to see things more clearly, notice and think about your available options, and decide what is best to do when you are grounded.

2. **Work to notice things that are different. Ask yourself: How is the here and now different than the past?**
   Strive to notice differences in situations, options, resources, people, and yourself. (This does not mean ignoring warning signs or minimizing things that are not OK. This means helping yourself notice when you actually *do* have options, resources, OK people, OK situations, and strengths that you did not have in the past so that you can make decisions with these in mind.)

3. **Continue to pay close attention to (and remind yourself of) the ways the present is different than the past.**
   This will help you keep the present separated from the past and stay more grounded. This helps you be better able to notice and think through what is best for you in the here and now.

TIPS: Remember that it is much easier to notice things that "fit" or agree with what we already believe or feel, so finding differences will require active effort and practice. Give yourself lots of credit when you are able to notice things you have not noticed before! (And, like all skills, keep practicing: The more you practice, the easier it will get, and the more it will help!)

---

[1] Loewenstein, 2006; Rothschild, 2000.

Why work to separate the past from the present?

Separating past from present helps you see the here and now more clearly, which helps keep you safer, makes it easier to stay grounded, and helps you heal.

Separating past from present keeps you safer:

- Seeing the present clearly increases your awareness of what is actually happening.
- Seeing the present clearly makes it more likely you are able to notice the options, choices, and resources available to you that can help you.
- Seeing the present clearly makes it less likely that you will make decisions that you regret later.
- Seeing the present clearly makes it more likely that you make decisions that will keep you safe and are appropriate for the situation.

Separating past from present makes it easier to stay grounded:

- Confusion between the past and the present can lead to feeling too much or too little.
- Confusion between the past and the present can lead to dissociation and other trauma symptoms.

Separating past from present helps you heal:

- Seeing the present clearly makes it possible to learn new skills to help yourself (and to notice what helps and what works)!
- Seeing the present clearly makes it possible to learn and use healthy ways of relating to yourself and others.
- Seeing the present clearly helps you notice when the present is safer than the past, which helps your brain and body heal. (If unsafe things are happening, please let a treatment provider know!)
- Seeing the present clearly makes it possible to notice when situations and people are actually OK, and to connect with OK people if you choose to.

EXERCISES FOR TOPIC 4: SEPARATING PAST FROM PRESENT: WHEN, HOW, WHY

We hope you are continuing to practice using grounding skills and giving yourself lots of credit for all the hard work you are doing!

Posttraumatic stress disorder (PTSD) can lead people who have experienced trauma to confuse the "here and now" with the "there and then." A flashback is the most extreme version of this, but confusion between past and present can also happen in other ways for people who have experienced trauma. In these cases, situations can feel just like traumatic situations from the past. This can happen because something in the present reminds you of the past, or because you are afraid that something painful that has happened is happening again.

These experiences can be very scary and confusing—and can lead to choices that do not fit the here and now. The good news: Looking for, paying close attention to, and reminding yourself of the ways the present is different than the past (i.e., "separating the past from the present") will help you manage and reduce these experiences, keep you safer, and help you heal.

How will this keep you safer? Separating the past from the present will help you be more aware of what is truly happening in the here and now, and the options and resources you have available. In most situations, you are likely to have more options, resources, situations that are OK, people that are OK, and personal strengths than you did in the past. Decisions you make with the present in mind are more likely to be healthy and appropriate. As we emphasized in the information sheet for Topic 4, separating past from present is not about minimizing things that are not OK. (Please talk to a treatment provider about any current situations or relationships that are not OK!) The goal is to help you notice when you *do* have options, resources, OK people, OK situations, and strengths that you did not have before. You do not want to ignore or minimize those—noticing these things helps you heal!

Separating past from present also helps you notice when you are safer, including times where you might be *feeling* danger from the past—or when something or someone *reminds* you of danger from the past—but you are thankfully *not in danger* in the present. Noticing when you are safer is an essential part of the healing process. Each moment you can actively notice that you are safer, if even for a moment, helps your brain and all of who you are heal.

This is why separating past from present is so important: When we do not clearly see what is happening in the here and now, we may unintentionally make choices that put our safety at risk or get in the way of our healing.

The exercises below focus on helping you notice differences between the past and present. As always, your safety comes first. Pay attention to warning signs (such as feeling too much or too little); take breaks if you need to; and use grounding skills if you start to feel too much or too little, get overwhelmed, or start to dissociate.

Written Exercises for Topic 4: Separating Past from Present: When, How, Why

Written exercise 1: Thinking mistakes that can make it harder to notice differences between the past and the present

It is hard to notice and pay attention to things that do not fit what we already think, believe, or feel. (The stronger we believe or feel something, the harder it can be to notice things that do not fit. This is why it is so important to give yourself credit when you notice things you have not before!) This difficulty can make it easy to make thinking mistakes.

Thinking mistakes can lead us to believe (or keep believing) things that are not true—and can get in the way of noticing differences between the past and the present. To help you become aware of thinking mistakes that we are *all* at risk of making—and that make separating past from present particularly difficult—please read the list of thinking mistakes in the table below.[2] (Note that there are many areas of overlap among the different kinds of thinking mistakes.)

As you read about the thinking mistakes, please:

- Mark the thinking mistakes you notice you have made, and
- See the "How to help yourself see things more clearly" column for suggestions on how to help yourself avoid making these mistakes.

Thinking mistakes that we're all at risk of making	Examples of these kinds of thinking mistakes	How to help yourself see things more clearly
All-or-nothing thinking: Seeing things in extremes	Seeing situations as either completely OK or not at all OK, completely safe or not safe at all, all good or all bad, perfect (or OK) or a disaster	Without minimizing, work to notice and pay attention to "the in-between"—for example, when situations are more OK, safer, or better. Please also notice what helps you recognize this.
Filtering out the positive/ magnifying the negative: Paying so much attention to negative details that all positive aspects of an experience are ignored and/or dismissed as not counting	Doing really well at something and getting positive feedback about it, but feeling like you are completely incompetent after someone points out you made a minor error	Remind yourself of the positive aspects so as not to minimize them. (In this example: Remind yourself what you *did* accomplish, and give yourself credit for that.)

---

[2] Informed by Beck, 1976; Boon et al., 2011, pp. 237–239; Burns, 2012; Leahy, 2017; Sheppard Pratt Health System Trauma Disorders Unit "Cognitive Distortions" overview, 2009.

Thinking mistakes that we're all at risk of making	Examples of these kinds of thinking mistakes	How to help yourself see things more clearly
Overgeneralizing: Assuming that something that is true of one situation (or several similar situations) will be true in all situations, no matter how different the situations are	Assuming that the way one person has responded to you will always be the way all people will respond	Remind yourself that different situations and people are different ("different people are different people"), and work to notice the details of the here and now so as not to miss differences.
Jumping to negative conclusions/predicting catastrophe: Having a strongly held belief about something without evidence	Assuming you did something wrong or are in trouble when you learn that someone wants to talk with you	Work to not minimize in either direction (try to not assume the worst or the best) and think about what else might happen. (In these examples: The other person might want to ask about something you know about, or to share good news.)
Mislabeling: Attaching an unfair label to a person, place, thing, or situation that is extreme and accompanied by strong emotion	After you make a single mistake or can't do something perfectly the first time, you think, "I am such a loser!" or "I will never be able to do this!"	Remind yourself to consider what is fair to expect. (In these examples: It is not fair to expect anyone to be perfect, and it takes time to learn new things. "I may not be able to do this the way I would like to *yet*, but if I keep practicing, I will get there!")

Written exercise 2: Noticing differences between the past and present

Practicing skills when you do not actively need them helps you be better prepared and more successful when you do need them. This exercise is focused on helping you notice differences in the present while you are as grounded as possible. This will make it easier for you to remind yourself of these differences when you need to, including when staying oriented to and anchored in the present is especially hard.

As always when doing work related to this program, please start by orienting and anchoring to the present to make sure you are grounded. This will help you think more clearly. Please pay attention to any signs you are starting to feel too much or too little and remember to pause and get grounded if you need to.

> *TIPS:* As you go through this exercise, be on the lookout for the understandable thinking errors we just described. If you are having a hard time identifying differences (especially improvements) in the here and now, review the thinking errors table again. See if you might be caught in one or more of them. (And be sure to give yourself lots of credit if you are able to notice this—this is hard work!)

Are you grounded? If yes, let's start with resources. What resources do you have now that you did not have then? (For example, in the here and now, do you have a safer place to live, safer access to money, safer access to the things you need?)

_____

_____

_____

_____

_____

Next, let's look at personal strengths. What personal strengths do you have now that you did not have then? (For example, do you know more ways to help yourself and/or get help now than in the past? Are you stronger? Better able to care for and take care of yourself? Better able to see different options you have? Better able to make choices you feel good about later?)

_____

_____

_____

_____

_____

Now let's look at people and relationships. Are the people around you more OK than some people were in the past? Do you have more say about which people you are around now? Are you more aware of OK people you can talk to if some people are not OK in the present? (For example, are you aware that you can talk to a treatment provider if people in your life now are not OK? Please do so if anyone in your life now is not OK.) Please be sure to list the OK people you know and the people you can reach out to for help.

_____

_____

_____

_____

_____

_____

Finally, consider: Are there other ways the present is (or are there any things that make the present be) safer, freer, more positive, and/or more hopeful that don't seem to fit in the options above? If yes, please list those here.

_____

_____

_____

_____

_____

_____

Practice Exercise for Topic 4: Separating Past from Present: When, How, Why

Please take a little time each day to:

- Practice separating past from present by following the steps described in the information sheet.
- Work to separate past from present as soon as you start to feel like the present is reminding you of the past.
- Review your written exercise answers to help your remember the strengths, options, and help you have available now and ways to avoid falling into thinking mistakes.

These steps will help you get better and better at separating the past from the present, staying grounded, and thinking through what is best for you in the here and now.

What if you are not sure if something is actually different?

If you are not sure whether something is different enough to really be different, keep paying close attention, and work to notice things that are different without minimizing warning signs. Do your best to be grounded before making any important decisions.

TIPS:

- Learning this skill takes active effort and lots of practice—and noticing differences between the past and present will get easier over time.

- When looking at the differences between the past and present, it is very important to be self-compassionate. Often, the feelings you have in these present-day situations are feelings that were not safe to feel or show earlier.

- Please do not shame yourself for feelings about things that happened in the past. Instead, please remember to give yourself lots of credit when you notice times that you can feel differently about the here and now.

References for Topic 4

Beck, A. T. (1976). *Cognitive therapies and emotional disorders.* New American Library.

Boon, S., Steele, K., & van der Hart, O. (2011). *Coping with trauma-related dissociation: Skills training for patients.* W. W. Norton & Company.

Burns, D. D. (2012). *Feeling good: The new mood therapy.* New American Library.

Leahy, R. L. (2017). *Cognitive therapy techniques, second edition: A practitioner's guide.* Guilford Press.

Loewenstein, R. J. (2006). DID 101: A hands-on clinical guide to the stabilization phase of dissociative identity disorder treatment. *Psychiatric Clinics of North America, 29*(1), 305–332.

Rothschild, B. (2000). *The body remembers: The psychophysiology of trauma and trauma treatment.* W. W. Norton & Company.

Trauma Disorders Program, Sheppard Pratt Health System—Orienting handouts, v. 2009.

USING IMAGERY TO HELP SEPARATE PAST FROM PRESENT

Information Sheet for Topic 5

Reminder: When should I start separating the past from the present?

As soon as you find yourself starting to feel like . . .

- A situation is "like" or "just like" something from the past, or
- Something from the past is going to happen again.

How do I use imagery to help separate the past from the present?

1. **Start as usual: Use grounding skills** to *orient* and *anchor* yourself in the present. It's always easier to see things more clearly, notice and think about your available options, and decide what is best to do when you are grounded.

2. **Help yourself notice differences between past and present with "split screen" imagery:**[3]
   - Imagine an old TV showing the past that is getting triggered *(maybe with the sound off, or in black and white, or slightly blurry to help you notice it is not happening now)* or a modern TV screen showing the present with a small corner of the TV showing the past. Do what works best for you.
   - Work hard to notice ways the present is different than the past.
   - Once you see the present more clearly, change the "past" channel to a soothing, peaceful image, or turn it off.

3. **Use "containment" imagery**[4] **to help keep the past separated from the present:** Visualize taking a DVD (or some other recording of data) with the complete story of your past trauma out of the player and putting it away in a container until you have developed healthy coping skills strong enough to help you work through what happened.

TIP: Practicing with images not related to trauma will make it easier to use imagery to separate past from present when you really need it. The more you practice, the easier and more helpful it will get!

---

[3] Spiegel, 1981.
[4] International Society for the Study of Trauma and Dissociation, 2011; Kluft, 1982, 1989.

EXERCISES FOR TOPIC 5: USING IMAGERY TO HELP SEPARATE PAST FROM PRESENT

Working to notice how the present is different than the past can make a meaningful difference in helping you get and stay grounded. Recognizing what is happening in the here and now also helps you make better, safer decisions, and helps you heal. We hope you have been practicing this crucial skill and are beginning to experience and notice the ways it helps. We also hope you are giving yourself credit if you are able to notice differences or thinking errors. These are important accomplishments! Stick with it; it will get easier and more effective as you practice!

Imagery techniques can be very helpful in separating past from present.[5] The exercises below are designed to help you develop imagery that works well for you.

Written Exercises for Topic 5: Using Imagery to Help Separate Past from Present

Written exercise 1: Developing your split screen imagery

You have probably seen some televisions that can show a split screen, a screen that is divided so that you can watch two different events at the same time. Many people find it helpful to use split screen imagery when feeling something was just like a painful past event. Using split screen imagery in these situations can help you notice differences between the past and the present.

There are multiple ways to use split screen imagery. See which of the options below appeal to you—and feel free to create your own ways to make split screen work for you. We recommend starting by practicing with nontraumatic images or memories, so you have practice using the skill before you use it with more difficult images/memories.

- Imagine a modern TV screen showing the present on most of the screen with a small corner of the TV showing the past. You might make the picture from the past very small, slightly blurry, and quieter (or completely muted) to help you notice it is not happening now. Then work to notice ways the here and now (the present image) is different from the there and then (the past image). Please also work to recognize OK options and resources that are available to you now.

  When you are done, fade the old picture out, reminding yourself that what happened then was long ago, and you are now working on recovery and creating a healthy life. Or change the channel to something soothing and peaceful. If you want, you can keep looking at the calm, peaceful picture; you can make it larger; and you can turn up the volume on the peaceful scene. The calming image could be your pet, a trusted friend, a place that you enjoyed visiting or would like to visit, your therapist, or whatever is calming for you. You might imagine letting the current-day, peaceful picture expand to take over the whole screen. That can symbolize how you are healing.

---

[5] Spiegel, 1981. Also discussed in International Society for the Study of Trauma and Dissociation, 2011; Sheppard Pratt Trauma Disorders Program Patient handouts, v. 2013; Vermilyea, 2013.

- Or imagine an old TV showing the past that is getting triggered, maybe with the sound low, or in black and white, or slightly blurry to help you notice it is not happening now. Work to notice differences between the here and now and the images on the old TV. When done, turn the volume and brightness down on the past picture and turn it off, or change the channel to something soothing/calming.

My split screen

Describe what *your* split-screen imagery looks like: What does your TV look like? (Old? Modern?) What kind of functions and controls does it have? How will you use these functions to help you separate past from present?

_____

_____

_____

_____

_____

_____

_____

_____

_____

_____

_____

_____

_____

Once you have finished, consider drawing your TV and its controls, or finding pictures of the TV and controls like the ones you imagined.

Written exercise 2: Developing your containment imagery

In the information sheet for Topic 5, we described visualizing removing a DVD (or some other kind of recording or data file) with the story of past trauma and putting it away in a safe container[6] until you have healthy coping skills strong enough to help you work through what happened. This is a form of containment imagery, or what is sometimes simply referred to as "containment."

With practice (starting with nontraumatic material), many find that containment imagery offers meaningful help in managing intrusive symptoms. The idea is to:

1. Notice what is manageable. (Possible examples: that these events are not happening now, that the present is different from the past.)
2. Visualize putting away overwhelming images, memories, information, thoughts, and/or feelings in a container until a time when you are able to safely deal with them.

Some people imagine putting overwhelming memories in a safe, a secure lock box, or a strong bank vault, and then closing the door and locking it tight. Others imagine putting the memories in a photo album with a lock and locking it. Still others find it helpful to imagine storing these memories in a container made of a healing material that resides in a place that is also soothing, so that healing can happen even when the memories are contained. Others find it helpful to create a physical containment box and write "headlines" (a couple of words)[7] on pieces of paper that they put in this box, or to have a containment notebook with a lock on it for writing down headlines of past situations and then folding over the page and locking the journal. Use what works best for you—and feel free to be creative if you find other imagery that appeals to you as a safe way to store upsetting memories!

My containment imagery

Describe *your* container in detail. What does it look like? What is it made of? Does it have any special properties? Where is it? And what kind of closure mechanism does it have to keep overwhelming thoughts or memories in it for safekeeping until a time that it is manageable to address them?

_____

_____

_____

---

[6] International Society for the Study of Trauma and Dissociation, 2011; Kluft, 1982, 1989.
[7] Loewenstein, 2006.

_____

_____

_____

_____

Practice Exercise for Topic 5: Using Imagery to Help Separate Past from Present

Congratulations on developing imagery to help you separate past from present! Although split screen and containment imagery can be very helpful, it takes practice to learn to use them well.

To build your ability to use these skills, please take some time each day to practice using split screen and containment imagery with neutral or positive images:

- Imagine putting neutral or positive images on a split screen, changing their size, and adjusting their volume and picture.
- Practice putting neutral or positive images into your container, and then unlock the container and get the neutral or positive image back out.

Practicing with neutral or positive images will make it easier to learn these skills. It will also help to make it easier to use these techniques with more upsetting images.

Please also continue to practice and use grounding and separating past from present (including reviewing your strengths, options, resources, and help you have available) as needed, and give yourself credit each time you do. Every time you use these skills helps you make progress toward getting and feeling safer!

References for Topic 5

International Society for the Study of Trauma and Dissociation (ISSTD). (2011). Guidelines for treating dissociative identity disorder in adults, third revision. *Journal of Trauma & Dissociation, 12,* 115–187. https://doi.org/10.1080/15299732.2011.537247

Kluft, R. P. (1982). Varieties of hypnotic interventions in the treatment of multiple personality. *American Journal of Clinical Hypnosis, 24,* 230–240.

Kluft, R. P. (1989). Playing for time: Temporizing techniques in the treatment of multiple personality disorder. *American Journal of Clinical Hypnosis, 32,* 2, 90–98.

Loewenstein, R. J. (2006). DID 101: A hands-on clinical guide to the stabilization phase of dissociative identity disorder treatment. *Psychiatric Clinics of North America, 29,* 305–332.

Spiegel, D. (1981). Vietnam grief work using hypnosis. *American Journal of Clinical Hypnosis, 24,* 33–40.

Trauma Disorders Program, Sheppard Pratt Health System—Patient handouts, v. 2013.

Vermilyea, E. G. (2013). *Growing beyond survival: A self-help toolkit for managing traumatic stress.* Sidran Institute.

SEPARATING PAST FROM PRESENT: MANAGING 90/10 REACTIONS

Information Sheet for Topic 6

What are 90/10 reactions?[8]

A 90/10 reaction is when you have a very strong/intense reaction to a current situation because it triggers feelings from a past situation.

How do I help myself manage 90/10 reactions?

When you have an intense/overwhelming feeling, before acting on it:

1. **Get grounded.** Use grounding skills to *orient* and *anchor* yourself in the present. It is always easier to see things more clearly, notice and think about your available options, and decide what is best to do when you are grounded.

2. **Get curious.** Ask yourself: Is something in the here and now reminding me of the past? If yes, work to notice things that are different in the present (i.e., *separate past from present*).

3. **Be compassionate with yourself.** If your feelings are being influenced by the past, OR if your feelings are (also) related to something not OK now, please do not shame yourself for feelings about things that have happened (or are happening). Consider what you would tell someone you care about if they were in the same situation. Try to be kind and take care of yourself in the same way.

4. **Think about which healthy option will best help you make progress toward having the life you would like to have.**

5. **Put that option into action.**

TIP: When faced with difficulty, please show yourself the same compassion and kindness you would show someone else you care about if they were in the same situation.

---

[8] Lewis et al., 2004.

EXERCISES FOR TOPIC 6: SEPARATING PAST FROM PRESENT: MANAGING 90/10 REACTIONS

We hope you have been working to notice how the present is different than the past, have been practicing the imagery techniques that can help with this, and are giving yourself credit when you are able to notice differences. These are important accomplishments! (Stick with it; these skills will become easier to use and more effective as you practice!) This difficult but important work makes a significant difference in getting and staying grounded, making healthy decisions, and noticing when you are safer. This helps your brain and all of who you are heal.

Separating the past from the present helps you recognize when you are *feeling* danger from the past but are *not* currently in danger. Using this skill helps you realize that intense emotions are sometimes more related to the past than the present.

In the information sheet for Topic 6, we talked about 90/10 reactions: reacting much more strongly to a current situation because it triggers feelings from a past situation. In these situations, most of the feeling (maybe as much as 90% of it) is related to the past, with only a small part of the feeling (maybe as little as 10%) in response to what is happening in the current situation. It is usually much easier to notice other people having 90/10 reactions than to recognize them in ourselves.

This week's exercises will focus on helping you recognize when you are having 90/10 reactions.[9] Please be patient and compassionate with yourself as you do this work. Often, the feelings you have in these present-day situations are feelings that were not safe to feel or show earlier. Please do not shame yourself for feelings about things that happened to you in the past. Instead, remember to give yourself credit when you are able to notice that you can feel differently about what is happening in the here and now.

Written Exercises for Topic 6: Separating Past from Present: Managing 90/10 Reactions

Written exercise 1: Helping yourself notice and think about past 90/10 reactions
It is always easier to notice that something was a 90/10 reaction after it has happened. With this in mind, think back: Are you aware of having had any 90/10 reactions?

If you can think of more than one, choose one that is less difficult for you to think about as you answer the following questions. (Once you get practice, it will be easier to work on more difficult 90/10 reactions.)

If you are having difficulty thinking of a time you may have had a 90/10 reaction, think back to a time when you had an intense emotional reaction. Ask yourself, "Is it possible that some of the intense feelings I was having were from the past?" "Were these feelings being triggered by

---

[9] Adapted from Lewis et al., 2004, pp. 40–41.

something that reminded me of the past?" If you think the answer may be yes, use this situation for the following questions.

As always, get yourself grounded before you start, and take breaks and use your list of healthy ways to get grounded if you start to feel too much, too little, get overwhelmed, or start to dissociate.

1. Identifying 90/10 triggers

This first question is focused on helping you identify what may have triggered the 90/10 reaction: What was happening just before the 90/10 reaction that might have reminded you of the past? As you do this, please work hard to keep yourself focused on the present. When thinking or writing about how something reminded you of the past, stick to headline descriptions such as "this reminded me of an unsafe situation from the past."

_____

_____

_____

_____

_____

_____

_____

_____

_____

2. Noticing differences (separating past from present)

Think of the ways the situation that led to a 90/10 reaction was different than the past. Try to list as many differences as possible. If you are having difficulty, review the list of thinking mistakes to see if you might be caught in one or more thinking mistakes. Please be patient with yourself as you do this, and be sure to give yourself credit for noticing differences and thinking errors—this is hard work!

_____

_____

_____

_____

_____

_____

_____

_____

_____

_____

3. Noticing patterns

See if you can think of any other 90/10 reactions you may have had. If you can think of more than one 90/10 reaction, are there any common themes or triggers across the situations? If yes, describe these here. If you notice patterns, you can help yourself better prepare for these situations (see #4, "Reducing Vulnerability," below). This work will help these situations become less difficult to deal with over time.

_____

_____

_____

_____

_____

_____

_____

_____

4. Reducing vulnerability

If you notice patterns in situations that lead to 90/10 reactions, are there aspects of the present that might be helpful to stay aware of but are hard to notice when you are triggered? For example, do you have strengths, resources, options, or other things that can help you deal with the current situation and the triggered feelings from the past that you tend to forget about in the moment?

Are there things you could change to make the present even more different than the past? If yes, list those here to help yourself keep these in mind.

_____

_____

_____

_____

_____

_____

_____

_____

_____

Practice Exercise for Topic 6: Separating Past from Present: Managing 90/10 Reactions

You have been practicing getting and keeping yourself grounded, separating the past from the present by compassionately noticing differences between the here and now and the there and then and using imagery techniques that help separate the past from the present. Each of these steps will reduce the likelihood of having 90/10 reactions and will help make these old feelings more manageable when they do emerge.

We now encourage you to build on that work by being curious about the possibility of having a 90/10 reaction anytime you notice having very strong feelings by practicing the steps described in the information sheet (summarized below).

When you have an intense/overwhelming feeling, before acting on it:

1. **Get grounded.**
2. **Get curious.** Ask yourself: Is something in the here and now reminding me of the past? If yes, work to notice things that are different in the present (i.e., *separate past from present*).
3. **Be compassionate with yourself.**

4. **Think about which healthy option will best help you make progress toward having the life you would like to have. Put that option into action.**

Recognizing 90/10 reactions leads to new, healthy pathways in your brain as you develop new understandings of yourself, your feelings, the present, and the past. You are healing and getting stronger and healthier each time you recognize a 90/10 reaction, so be sure to give yourself credit for making progress each time you do!

TIPS:

- When faced with difficulty, please show yourself the same compassion and kindness you would show someone else you care about in the same situation.
- Remember to practice grounding when you don't need it, and to use grounding when you first notice signs of feeling too much or too little to help yourself stay grounded and thinking clearly.
- If something feels like or reminds you of something from the past, work to notice how the present situation and your present options and resources are different. This will help you be better able to notice and think through what is best for you in the here and now.
- If aspects of the past have been triggered, remember that you can use *containment imagery*. Imagine putting those parts of the past into some type of container, like a very strong bank vault or a solid, secure box that you can "open" later, when you are ready to. This can help you feel a distance from the past. Then use grounding skills to get anchored back in present reality before going on about your day. If you were really shaken, it can take a while to do this. Start with something from your list of healthy ways to help yourself when feeling too much or too little.
- Consider talking about 90/10 reactions with a treatment provider.
- Once you have enough distance from strong emotions, consider using the questions and exercises in this topic to help you manage other 90/10 reactions.

Congratulations on completing the second module! The work you've begun in these first two modules will serve as a foundation for the rest of the work we'll be doing in this program. Working to keep yourself grounded and separating the past from the present will go a long way toward helping you get and feel safer.

In the modules that follow, we'll offer additional skills that will help you make progress toward getting and feeling safer. Step by step, you'll get there!

Reference for Topic 6

Lewis, L., Kelly, K., & Allen, J. (2004). *Restoring hope and trust: An illustrated guide to mastering trauma.* Sidran Institute Press.

MODULE 3

Additional Foundations

Grounding and separating past from present are core foundations for managing and reducing trauma-related symptoms. Using them as needed will go a long way toward helping you heal— and toward getting the most out of the rest of this program.

This module offers additional ways to help you make progress toward getting and feeling safer as you prepare to work through the rest of this program.

This module will help you learn:

- more healthy ways to help when you're feeling too much
- things you can do toward healing the impact of trauma
- steps you can expect along the way toward healing
- how to help yourself manage crisis-level feelings
- how to help yourself make the best progress in the healing process
- signs you might be having trauma-related thoughts, and steps to manage them.

This module will help you practice:

- developing and using imagery techniques for when you're feeling too much
- approaching the healing process in ways that are most likely to help
- developing and using plans for managing intense emotions
- noticing and managing trauma-based thoughts.

This work will help you make additional progress toward getting and feeling safer. This work will also serve as a bridge to the rest of the work you will be doing in this program.

MORE HEALTHY WAYS TO HELP YOURSELF WHEN YOU'RE FEELING TOO MUCH

Information Sheet for Topic 7

Deep breathing

Deep breathing *(belly breathing)* can be a powerful means of helping yourself when you're feeling too much.

Take a long, deep breath—the kind of breath that makes your belly rise. Then exhale fully, letting go of stress and worry. Breathe in again, taking a slow, deep breath, and then let it go, too, taking stress and worry with it.

With each breath, allow your mind to focus on your breathing. Slowly breathing in, slowly breathing out, notice as your mind and body become quieter and more focused on the here and now. Remind yourself to breathe deeply as necessary.

- *TIP 1:* If you notice yourself beginning to think about things other than your breathing while you're doing this, remind yourself to breathe deeply, and bring your focus back to your breathing. ("Mind wandering" is normal, especially early in the process of learning how to do this!)
- *TIP 2:* Deep breathing also helps you get and stay grounded. (When we don't get deep breaths, our bodies think something bad might be happening—so make sure to take slow, deep breaths if you start to feel too much!)

Slow swing

Imagine yourself on a swing, slowly swinging up, then down; up, then down. As you do, notice what it feels like to be going back and forth, feeling the breeze as you do.

- *TIP:* If deep breathing is hard for you, this is a great alternative!

Peaceful place imagery

Think of a beautiful, relaxing, soothing place you've been, read about, seen, or imagined—a place where you can feel yourself begin to relax just by thinking about it. Describe the setting to yourself in detail. What are you seeing? Hearing? Smelling? What is the light like? The temperature? The air?

- *TIP 1:* Consider thinking about a peaceful place[1] where you have all you need to feel OK, protected, and maybe even happy. Where is it? What's there?
- *TIP 2:* If deep breathing is hard for you, consider imagining a swing in a peaceful place and using "Slow Swing" (above).

Gauges

Imagery can also be used to help you notice how you are doing. *Gauges*[2] can help you notice and be aware of the intensity of your impulses or level of distress and the need to seek out help.

Gauges come in multiple forms. For example,

- *Thermometers* can help you know when things are getting "too hot."
- *Pressure gauges* can let you know when internal pressure is getting "too high."
- *Speedometers* can help you know when things are moving "too fast."
- *A series of colors* can indicate levels of risk of impulsive action. (For example: blue = calm, green = OK, yellow = slightly elevated risk, orange = increased risk, and red = danger.)

Regulators

Visualizing *regulators*[3] can help you adjust the levels of different aspects of your experience. For example:

- You could use a *control knob*, *dial*, *variable switch*, or *lever* to turn down overwhelming emotions.
- You could use a *control knob* or *dial* to reduce the intensity of impulses, anxiety, or memories of the past.
- You could use a *lever* or *brake pedal* to slow the speed of racing thoughts.
- You can also use *dials* and *levers* to turn up the awareness of different aspects of the safe present.

---

[1] Hammond, 1990; Kluft, 1982, 1989.
[2] Trauma Disorders Program, Sheppard Pratt, 2013; Vermilyea, 2013.
[3] Daitch, 2007; Hammond, 1990; Trauma Disorders Program, Sheppard Pratt, 2013; Vermilyea, 2013.

The pause button

Using a pause button[4] can be a great way to give yourself time to think things through before making any decisions that you might regret later. This can be especially helpful when you are feeling intense urges or impulses to do something before thinking though what is most likely to help you make progress toward having the kind of life you want. One way of approaching this is to tell yourself, "When I start to get overwhelmed, I'll push the pause button and get grounded before deciding what to do."

---

[4] Lewis et al., 2004.

EXERCISES FOR TOPIC 7: MORE HEALTHY WAYS TO HELP YOURSELF WHEN YOU'RE FEELING TOO MUCH

We hope you have been working to notice times that you might be having 90/10 reactions and are giving yourself credit when you are able to notice that this is the case. Realizing when intense emotions are related to the past is an important accomplishment!

The information sheet for Topic 7 presented more healthy ways to help yourself when you are feeling too much. To help you personalize the imagery techniques we talked about, the next written exercises focus on helping you develop your own peaceful place imagery, gauges, and regulators.

Imagery involves using the imagination. We use our imagination for all kinds of tasks, and what we imagine strongly influences how we feel. For example, when we imagine being in a place that feels peaceful and safer, we begin to feel more and more of what it feels like to be there. With this in mind, let's talk about peaceful place imagery.

Written Exercises for Topic 7: More Healthy Ways to Help Yourself When You're Feeling Too Much

Written exercise 1: Developing peaceful place imagery
Many people find peaceful place imagery helpful in addressing emotional overwhelm (feeling too much).

Think of the most beautiful, relaxing, soothing place(s) you have been, seen pictures of, read about, or imagined—places where you can feel yourself begin to relax just by thinking about them. In a moment, we will ask you to describe it.

Notes:

- Some people may find it anxiety-provoking to even consider relaxing. If you begin to feel more anxious as you think about relaxing, you might find it more useful to imagine a place that is "more OK" or "more peaceful." We encourage anyone with concerns about imagery to talk to a treatment provider to determine the best way to deal with their concerns.
- For people who have parts: If a part of you is concerned about participating in this exercise, we recommend that this part observe this exercise to see how it goes. We encourage any part of you that is not going to participate in this exercise to allow other parts to participate or watch. Perhaps that concerned part is having trauma-based thoughts and needs to see if it is OK and safe to use imagery.

Your peaceful place(s)
Think about the most beautiful, relaxing, soothing place you have been, seen pictures of, read about, or imagined. Describe it in detail below.

(For example: What place[s] help you feel a bit more relaxed just by thinking about them? What do you see there? What do you hear? What is the air/temperature like? Are there any smells there? If yes, describe those, too.)

_____

_____

_____

_____

_____

_____

_____

_____

_____

_____

_____

_____

Think of colors, things, situations that make you feel more calm, protected, and safe. List those here:

_____

_____

_____

———————————————————

———————————————————

———————————————————

———————————————————

———————————————————

Now imagine a place and situation that is safe (or safer, or more peaceful, or whatever description sounds most healing to you) and perfectly attuned to your preferences. This is a place where you have all you need to feel OK, protected, and maybe even happy.

Describe the setting in detail. *(What are you seeing? Hearing? What is the light like? The temperature? Any smells? What do you have there that helps you feel more protected, safe, or happy? What colors do you notice?)*

Did more than one scenario come to mind? If so, that is wonderful! Describe each of them.

———————————————————

———————————————————

———————————————————

———————————————————

———————————————————

———————————————————

———————————————————

———————————————————

———————————————————

———————————————————

———————————————————

_____

_____

_____

_____

_____

_____

_____

TIPS:

- To improve your ability to visualize your peaceful place imagery, consider drawing or cutting out pictures representing the places, colors, things, and situations you listed. Some people find it helpful to carry small objects that remind them of their peaceful places. (For example, they may select a shell if their peaceful place is a beach.)

- If you have parts, invite each of your parts to follow the same process—all parts of you deserve peaceful places, places where each part of you feels safe, peaceful, and/or comfortable, and where you have things around you that bring you comfort! Each part that is willing to participate in this exercise can choose if they would like to be in a shared place with other parts, or if they would prefer having their own place.

Written exercise 2: Developing gauges and regulators

As we discussed in the information sheet for Topic 7, gauge and regulator imagery can be used to help you notice how you are doing and manage overwhelming feelings and intrusive images and thoughts. This exercise will invite you to think about how you might like to use gauges and regulators.

Notice which forms work most well and naturally for you. Incorporate the imagery that you find useful into your list of coping skills.

Visualizing *gauges* can help you be aware of the intensity of impulses or your level of distress and the need to seek out help. Gauges come in multiple forms. For example:

- *Thermometers* can help you know when things are getting "too hot."
- *Pressure gauges* can let you know when internal pressure is getting "too high."

- *Speedometers* can help you know when things are moving "too fast."
- A *series of colors* can indicate levels of safety vs. risk of impulsive action (for example: blue = calm, green = OK, yellow = slightly elevated risk, orange = increased risk, and red = danger).

Use this space to write about the kinds of gauge imagery you would like to use, and how you will use this imagery:

_____

_____

_____

_____

_____

_____

_____

Regulators can help you adjust the levels of different aspects of your experience. For example, you can use:

- A *control knob, dial, variable switch,* or *lever* to turn down overwhelming emotions;
- A *control knob* or *dial* to reduce the intensity of impulses, anxiety, or memories of the past;
- A *lever* or *brake pedal* to slow the speed of racing thoughts; or
- *Dials* and *levers* to turn up the awareness of different aspects of the safe present.

Use this space to write about the kinds of regulator imagery you would like to use, and how you will use this imagery:

_____

_____

_____

_____

_____

_____

_____

_____

_____

Congratulations on developing gauge and regulator imagery!

TIP: To improve your ability to visualize your gauge and regulator imagery, you may find it helpful to draw or find images that reflect what your gauges and regulators look like.

Written exercise 3: The pause button

The *pause button* is another helpful form of imagery. We have talked about using regulators (like levers, or maybe a brake pedal) to slow things down. Using a pause button can be a great way to help give yourself time to think about things before making any decisions that you might regret later.

This can be helpful when you notice yourself beginning to feel overwhelmed, or notice that you are at risk of doing something that is not healthy.

You could tell yourself, "When I start to get overwhelmed, I will push the pause button and review my list of healthy ways to help myself when feeling too much or too little."

Imagine this kind of pause button. What does it look like? How can you help yourself remember to use it?

_____

_____

_____

_____

_____

_____

_____

_____

_____

_____

_____

Practice Exercise for Topic 7: More Healthy Ways to Help Yourself When You're Feeling Too Much

Deep breathing, peaceful places, slow swing, gauges, and regulators can each be very helpful; like all skills, however, it takes practice to learn to use them well.

To build your ability to use these skills, please take some time each day to practice using them. Because using these skills effectively takes practice, we encourage you to practice them and use them before you need to. We also encourage you to add them to your list of healthy ways to help yourself when you are feeling too much or too little.

Please also continue to practice and use grounding and separating past from present. Give yourself credit each time you do. Every time you use these skills helps you make progress toward getting and feeling safer!

References for Topic 7

Daitch, C. (2007). *Affect regulation toolbox: Practical and effective hypnotic interventions for the over-reactive client.* Norton.

Hammond, D. C. (1990). *Handbook of hypnotic suggestions and metaphors.* Norton.

Kluft, R. P. (1982). Varieties of hypnotic interventions in the treatment of multiple personality. *American Journal of Clinical Hypnosis, 24,* 230–240.

Kluft, R. P. (1989). Playing for time: Temporizing techniques in the treatment of multiple personality disorder. *American Journal of Clinical Hypnosis, 32,* 2, 90–98.

Lewis, L., Kelly, K., & Allen, J. (2004). *Restoring hope and trust: An illustrated guide to mastering trauma.* Sidran Institute Press.

Trauma Disorders Program, Sheppard Pratt Health System—Patient handouts, v. 2013.

Vermilyea, E. G. (2013). *Growing beyond survival: A self-help toolkit for managing traumatic stress.* Sidran Institute.

HOW TO HELP YOURSELF HEAL THE IMPACT OF TRAUMA ON THE BRAIN

Information Sheet for Topic 8

Trauma significantly impacts your brain's default responses. This can make it much harder to not get overwhelmed. **Practicing healthy coping helps our brains** (and all of who we are) **heal.**

How does trauma impact the brain?

Trauma activates and strengthens fear pathways, making them overactive and overdeveloped.

- As part of the brain's effort to protect against further harm, traumatized brains become highly sensitive to even the slightest signs of possible danger.

- In dangerous situations, overdeveloped fear pathways can be life-saving—they can literally help a person survive in a dangerous environment.

- However, once someone is no longer in a dangerous situation, their fear pathways can stay hyperalert to potential threats. This is why people who have been traumatized can feel threatened so often. This is also what can keep people feeling highly unsafe and having trauma-related reactions in safer situations.

- The brain also provides an escape from overwhelming situations: dissociation. When someone dissociates, the emotional parts of the brain shut down. In frightening situations, dissociation helps the world feel less real or overwhelming, and can help a person get through otherwise unbearable situations.

- *BUT:* If dissociation continues when situations are safer, people may not learn to tolerate emotions and normal body sensations. Instead, they may get in the habit of tuning these out. Eventually, it may be difficult for the person to realize when they are hungry, full, sleepy, getting sick, or feeling an emotion.

- Not feeling feelings and body sensations can be dangerous. What if someone or something is truly wrong in the present, and a person does not feel the feelings that could tell them this? For example, what if they are ill but cannot feel their body well enough to know this? They would not know that they need to get to the doctor.

- So the very reactions that help people survive during trauma may later become habits that make it difficult to heal, recover, and be healthy.

Using healthy recovery-focused skills (like the ones in this program) helps your brain:

- understand when you are safer
- build new, calm, healthy pathways
- reduce activation of fear pathways when situations are safer.

Each effort you make (whether you notice or not!) helps toward your goal!

What are the steps I can expect along the way toward healing and recovery?

Research looking at the process of therapeutic change has found that people go through a predictable series of steps/stages along the way.[5]

More specifically, people typically move from:

- being **unaware** of a problem, to
- **actively avoiding** thoughts and situations that remind of the problem;
- being **vaguely aware** that there might be a problem;
- **clarifying** the problem ("I think the problem is that . . .");
- **empathically understanding** the problem ("Oh . . . THAT's why this is like this"), which helps in
- applying what is understood to **work through the problem** (which often takes lots of practice!), which leads to
- increasingly being able to **resolve** the problem when it comes up; and
- ultimately (with even more practice) being able to **effectively respond** to situations that were once problematic.

TIPS:

- The early stages (and earliest parts of each stage) are often the hardest.
  Although changing how we do things almost always involves hard work, things do get easier and better as you go along. Keep practicing healthy, recovery-focused coping— you'll get there!

---

[5] Schielke et al., 2011; Stiles, 2011.

- Each of these steps reflects progress toward resolving the problem. Healing and recovery take lots of hard work, so it's important to give yourself credit for each milestone along the way!

For example: If you are becoming aware that you are having a problem staying grounded, give yourself credit for noticing that! If you are trying to get better at using grounding skills as soon as you notice signs of getting ungrounded, give yourself credit each time you are able to notice yourself getting ungrounded—EVEN IF you are not yet always able to use grounding skills when you need them. Give yourself credit each time you practice a skill when you don't need it, each time you try to use a skill when you do need it, and each time you are able to use a skill to help yourself get grounded. These are important accomplishments.

EXERCISES FOR TOPIC 8: HOW TO HELP YOURSELF HEAL THE IMPACT OF TRAUMA ON THE BRAIN

We hope you have been practicing using deep breathing and/or imagery techniques and have begun to find them helpful.

The information sheet for Topic 8 focused on how to help you heal from trauma's impact on the brain, including an overview of the process people go through when working toward solving a problem.

Learning how to do things differently takes repeated practice. As you work to create new habits, please notice and give yourself credit for each bit of progress. And remember—the more you practice skills when you don't urgently need them, the more you will be able to use them when you really do need them.

The exercises below will help you think about how to apply what you have been learning.

Written Exercises for Topic 8: How to Help Yourself Heal the Impact of Trauma on the Brain

Written exercise 1: Planning which healthy coping skills to use when
Learning about something that can be helpful to do (like a new coping skill) makes it possible to begin to put that information into practice. Even so, it can be hard to remember to do things differently without a specific plan for when and how you are going to use the new skills you have learned.

In this exercise, we invite you to think about when and how you can use healthy coping skills that you know or are in the process of learning, starting with the healing-focused coping skills we have been introducing as part of this program. Use the table that follows to plan when and how you'll use healthy coping skills to help yourself. *(Note: We have left a number of blank "healthy coping skill" spaces for planning when and how to use any other healthy skills you find helpful.)*

Healthy coping skill	When/how I will use it
Grounding *(orienting to/anchoring in the present)*	
Separating past from present	
Split screen imagery	
Containment imagery	
Deep breathing	
Slow swing imagery	
Peaceful place imagery	

Healthy coping skill	When/how I will use it
Gauge imagery	
Regulator imagery	
The pause button	

Practice Exercise for Topic 8: How to Help Yourself Heal the Impact of Trauma on the Brain

To help yourself heal, we encourage you to practice using healthy ways of coping. Making plans for difficult situations will help: Planning ahead makes it more likely that you will be able to help yourself interrupt the process of getting overwhelmed and cope in a healthy way.

It may be helpful to know that, when practicing doing something differently, people tend to go through these steps over time:

- First, we tend to realize what we could have done (e.g., which coping skill we could have used) *after* the situation is over.
- Later, we notice what we can do *while* the problem situation is happening, but have difficulty doing the new thing.
- Eventually, we realize what we could do *before* the situation gets problematic, but have difficulty doing the new thing, and then . . .

- Ultimately, with practice, we're able to recognize what we can do before the problem happens *and* be able to do the new thing, initially with a lot of difficulty—and then it becomes easier as we get more practice!

  And remember: Each of these steps reflects progress toward resolving the problem.

Please be patient and compassionate with yourself as you go through the process of learning to use these skills when you need them, reminding yourself that learning how to do things differently takes time and repeated practice. And don't forget to notice and give yourself credit for each bit of progress along the way—each step toward healing makes a difference in helping your brain (and all of who you are) heal!

References for Topic 8

Schielke, H. J., Stiles, W. B., Cuellar, R. E., Fishman, J. L., Hoener, C., Del Castillo, D., Dye, A. K., Zerubavel, N., Walker, D. P., & Greenberg, L. S. (2011). A case study investigating whether the process of resolving interpersonal problems in couple therapy is isomorphic to the process of resolving problems in individual therapy. *Pragmatic Case Studies in Psychotherapy, 7*, 477–528. doi:10.14713/pcsp.v7i4.1114

Stiles, W. B. (2011). Coming to terms. *Psychotherapy Research, 21*, 367–384. doi:10.1080/10503307.2011.582186

MANAGING CRISIS-LEVEL FEELINGS

Information Sheet for Topic 9

Reminders of trauma can trigger powerful feelings that can become overwhelming. Intense feelings can make it seem like an emergency is happening. These kinds of situations can be difficult to manage with only one coping skill. Think about how to combine the healthy skills that work for you to help you manage these situations in healthy ways.

How do I manage crisis-level feelings?

Here is one way to use the strategies we have talked about in this program to help you manage crisis-level feelings:

1. **Hit the "pause" button.** Then . . .
2. **Breathe.** Do some deep breathing to calm your mind. While you do . . .
3. **Get grounded.** Use grounding skills to orient yourself to and anchor yourself in the present.
4. **Separate past from present and manage trauma-based thoughts.** Remind yourself of the resources, strengths, and healthy options you have in the here and now. Use "split screen" to notice differences between past and present.
5. **Dial down triggering material from the past.** Use regulator imagery to turn down images, thoughts, or feelings related to the past.
6. **Contain overwhelming images, thoughts, and emotions.** Containment imagery can help you put away anything from the past that has been triggered. You might imagine that you are putting old memories, images, feelings, sensations, sights, smells—or anything else that gets triggered from past traumas—in a container, like a safe, until you are able to manage them safely.
7. **Remind yourself—all of you—that feelings come and go.** Even when feelings are very strong, they eventually pass. It can be helpful to remember that you have already survived many very challenging things. Use peaceful place imagery or distract yourself with pleasant, safe activities, such as listening to soothing music, until the feelings pass.
8. **Give yourself the care you need.** Follow your healthy coping plan as you need to when feeling too much or too little.
9. **Approach this work with healthy self-compassion.** Changing how you do things takes lots of practice over time. Step by step, you'll get there!

EXERCISES FOR TOPIC 9: MANAGING CRISIS-LEVEL FEELINGS

We hope you have been practicing using healthy coping skills and following your healthy coping plan. We also hope you are striving to be patient and compassionate with yourself as you learn to use these skills. Remind yourself that learning how to do things differently takes time and repeated practice. Please notice and give yourself credit for each bit of progress along the way.

In the information sheet for Topic 9, we talked about managing crisis-level feelings—intense feelings that can make it feel like an emergency is happening. Please review the information sheet before continuing on to the exercises below, which focus on helping you identify healing-focused ways to manage these kinds of feelings.

Written Exercise for Topic 9: Managing Crisis-Level Feelings

Developing a plan to manage crisis-level feelings
In the information sheet for Topic 9, we emphasized the importance of using safety/healthy coping plans to help you manage these times in healthy ways. Managing crisis-level feelings with healing-focused coping skills—like the ones introduced in this program—helps slow and reduce the cycle of feeling too much or too little, feeling unsafe, and unhealthy behavior.

Crisis-level feelings are more likely to be safely managed through the use of a combination of skills, with each skill addressing different parts of the problem. The information sheet offered one way to combine the use of the techniques introduced in this program to manage crisis-level feelings.

This exercise will encourage you to reflect on what combination of skills might be most helpful for you when experiencing crisis-level feelings. As with all work on this program, make sure you are grounded before beginning this work, and take breaks to ground if you start to feel too much or too little. Our goal is for you to get and feel safer—please put safety and healthy coping first.

Are you grounded? Let's start by making a list of healthy coping skills that *you* have found helpful.

Healthy coping skills that I have found helpful:

_____

_____

_____

_____

_____

_____

_____

_____

_____

_____

_____

_____

_____

_____

Now, consider how you might combine those skills to help yourself manage crisis-level feelings well. (If the information sheet's suggestions feel helpful, please feel free to use as many of them as you like!)

How I will combine the healthy coping skills I have found helpful to manage crisis-level feelings:

_____

_____

_____

_____

_____

_____

_____

_____

_____

_____

_____

_____

_____

_____

_____

_____

Practice Exercise for Topic 9: Managing Crisis-Level Feelings

Congratulations on developing a plan to manage crisis-level feelings!

We encourage you to continue to practice using healthy coping skills, to follow your healthy coping plan, and to review and practice your new plan for managing crisis-level feelings. We encourage you to be patient and compassionate with yourself as you learn to use these skills. Remind yourself that learning how to do things differently takes time and repeated practice.

TIPS:

When practicing doing something differently, people tend to go through these steps over time:

- First, we tend to realize what we could have done (e.g., which coping skill we could have used) *after* the situation is over.
- Later, we notice what we can do *while* the problem situation is happening, but have difficulty doing the new thing.
- Eventually, we realize what we could do *before* the situation gets problematic, but have difficulty doing the new thing, and then . . .
- Ultimately, with practice, we're able to recognize what we can do before the problem happens *and* be able to do the new thing, initially with a lot of difficulty—and then it becomes easier as we get more practice!

Don't forget to give yourself credit for all the work you are doing and each bit of progress along the way! Each effort you make helps your brain (and all of who you are) heal.

Step by step, you will get there!

THE IMPORTANCE OF SELF-COMPASSION IN THE HEALING PROCESS

Information Sheet for Topic 10

Taking care of yourself in healthy ways will help your brain, body, and all of who you are get and feel safer. To best help yourself manage difficult situations in healthy ways, **please be compassionate with yourself when you are going through difficult times.**

Why is compassion so important in the healing process?

Being gentle, fair, and encouraging makes it easier to understand and resolve problems by:
- reducing the likelihood of overwhelming emotions
- making it easier to find good solutions
- making it easier to stick with the process of learning/practicing new ways of doing things.

How does harsh criticism get in the way of healing?

Being harshly critical of yourself is likely to increase your difficulties. "Beating yourself up" with harsh criticism and/or shaming yourself:
- makes you feel badly about yourself
- drains you of energy you need to make healthy changes, and
- can make you feel like you do not deserve to be healthy or safe.

Being uncaring does not help—it hurts

- *Minimizing or ignoring something true does not work.* Ignoring things that are true gets in the way of finding solutions for problems that work well for everyone.
- *Minimizing or ignoring feelings does not work.* It does not feel good to be told what we are thinking or feeling is not important—in fact, this is more likely to make us more upset.

How do I get better at being compassionate with myself?

- Think about what you would tell a child or adult you care deeply about if they were in your exact same situation. If something is true for someone else, it is only fair for it to be true for you, too.
- Give yourself compassion by using the "GIVE" skill[6] with yourself. Be:
  - *Gentle:* We all do better when we are treated with gentle care.
  - *Interested:* Be interested in and curious about what is happening.
  - *Validating:* Acknowledge and validate (not minimize) what is true, and do this in an
  - *Easy mannered:* Use self-talk that is calming and encouraging, even if you're not able to do things exactly as you wish yet.

It is compassionate to show you care

One way to help remember how to show yourself care. Be . . .

- *Curious* about what can help you.
- *Acknowledge* context (i.e., things that are influencing your current situation). For example: "My trauma-related reactions make sense given my trauma experiences" or "It takes lots of practice to be able to do things in new ways."
- *Reflect* on options before acting: Which option will best help you make progress toward healing and recovery (getting and feeling safer)?
- *Encourage* yourself to put that option into practice, even (and especially!) when you do not feel able to take a healthy step.

TIPS:

- Please be patient with yourself as you work to give yourself the care you need; changing how you relate to yourself takes lots of practice.
- Working to be compassionate with yourself while you are learning to be more self-compassionate can be difficult—and is a powerful way to make progress.
- It is important to give yourself credit for each step along the way. For example: Since it is hard to notice when we are not being compassionate with ourselves, be sure to give yourself credit every time you are able to notice you are being harsh or not self-compassionate—and every time you make progress in giving care to yourself.

---

[6] Adapted with permission from Guilford Press. Interpersonal Effectiveness Handout 6, pg. 128. Linehan, M. (2015). DBT skills training handouts and worksheets, second edition. New York: The Guilford Press.
[Linehan, M. (2015). DBT skills training handouts and worksheets, second edition. New York: The Guilford Press.].

EXERCISES FOR TOPIC 10: THE IMPORTANCE OF SELF-COMPASSION IN THE HEALING PROCESS

We hope you have been practicing using healthy coping skills and noticing and giving yourself credit for each bit of progress along the way.

In the information sheet for Topic 10, we emphasized that an important part of helping yourself is not just *what* you do, but *how* you do it. More specifically, we talked about how self-compassion makes it easier to do the things that help you heal, and how minimizing, ignoring, and being harshly critical of yourself actually get in the way of getting and feeling safer.

It takes practice to change how you relate to yourself, though. Like anything else, it is easier to practice showing compassion to yourself when you are not overwhelmed than when you are already feeling too much or too little. With this in mind, the exercises below focus on helping you identify ways to be compassionate with yourself.

Written Exercise for Topic 10: The Importance of Self-Compassion in the Healing Process

Identifying ways to increase your self-compassion

To help remember how to be compassionate with yourself, we suggested you GIVE yourself care by being:

- **Gentle:** We all do better when we are treated with gentle care.
- **Interested:** Be interested in and curious about what is happening, being especially curious about what you might not have noticed yet. (For example, you might notice that something is reminding you of the past; that you hadn't noticed how the current situation is different than the past; that you have more options and resources than you originally noticed.)
- **Validating:** Acknowledge and validate what is true without minimizing in any direction. (For example, "It makes sense that this is reminding me of the past and that this is difficult— and thankfully, this situation is different, and I have more resources and options now.")
- **Easy mannered:** Use self-talk that is calming and encouraging. (For example, it's important to give yourself credit for making progress any time you're able to notice something you originally missed—this is an accomplishment!)

We also suggested that you can show yourself compassionate CARE by remembering to be . . .

- **Curious** about what will help you.
- **Acknowledge** context—that is, the aspects of your life (past and present) that understandably contribute to your struggles. (For example, "My trauma-related reactions make sense given my trauma experiences" or "Being able to respond to challenging situations in new ways takes lots of practice.")

- ***Reflect*** on the skills you're learning and the options you have before deciding on your course of action. This will help you determine which option will best help you make progress toward your healing and recovery (getting and feeling safer).
- ***Encourage*** yourself to put that option into practice even (and especially) when you do not feel able to take a healthy step.

In the prompts below, we encourage you to think about ways you can be compassionate with yourself.

TIP: If you find yourself having difficulty thinking of options, think about what you would do for (or recommend to) a child or adult you care deeply about if they were in your exact same situation. Remember that if something is true for someone else, it is only fair for it to be true for you, too.

Gentle: What are some things you can do to be gentle with yourself?

_____

_____

_____

_____

_____

_____

_____

_____

_____

_____

_____

Interested: What are some things you can do that show interest in what you are experiencing and how you are doing? What could help you remember to look for things you haven't noticed yet (i.e., things that don't fit your interpretation of what is happening)?

_____

_____

_____

_____

_____

_____

_____

Validating: What can you do to help yourself acknowledge and validate what is true?

_____

_____

_____

_____

_____

_____

_____

Easy mannered: What can you do to help yourself remember to be fair and encouraging to yourself, even if you are not able to do things exactly as you wish yet?

_____

_____

_____

_____

_____

_____

_____

_____

__*Curious:*__ How can you help yourself remember to be curious about what will help?

_____

_____

_____

_____

_____

_____

_____

__*Acknowledge:*__ What can you do to help yourself remember to keep the context of what is happening in mind (e.g., "Trauma-related reactions make sense given a trauma history" or "It takes lots of practice to be able to do things in new ways")?

_____

_____

_____

_____

_____

_____

_____

_____

Reflect: How can you help yourself remember to consider your current resources and options and think about what will best help you make progress toward healing and recovery (getting and feeling safer)?

_____

_____

_____

_____

_____

_____

_____

Encourage: How can you help yourself remember to encourage yourself to do the things that will best help you make progress towards healing and recovery (getting and feeling safer)—especially when things are particularly difficult?

_____

_____

_____

_____

_____

_____

_____

_____

_____

_____

Practice Exercise for Topic 10: The Importance of Self-Compassion in the Healing Process

We encourage you to practice being compassionate with yourself (giving yourself the care you need) using the ideas of GIVE and CARE, especially when things are challenging. Please be patient with yourself as you go through the process of learning to use these skills, reminding yourself that changing how you relate to yourself takes lots of practice.

Working to be compassionate with yourself while you are learning to be more self-compassionate can be difficult—and is a powerful way to make progress. Don't forget to notice and give yourself credit for each bit of progress along the way—each effort makes a difference in helping your brain (and all of who you are) heal.

Step by step, you will get there!

Reference for Topic 10

Linehan, M. (2015). *DBT skills training handouts and worksheets* (2nd ed.). Guilford Press.

MANAGING TRAUMA-BASED THOUGHTS

Information Sheet for Topic 11

People who have experienced trauma often have trauma-based beliefs about themselves, others, and the world. Having these kinds of thoughts after experiencing trauma is understandable—they may have kept you safer then—and can make it difficult to notice when you are safer and have healthy options in the here and now.

What should I know about trauma-based thoughts?

- Trauma-based thoughts are a common trauma-related symptom. *(If you have them, it is not your fault.)*
- To help yourself heal, is important to help yourself notice the evidence against trauma-based thoughts *without minimizing that there are understandable reasons why you are having such thoughts.*
- Noticing evidence against trauma-based thoughts takes lots of active effort and practice.
- This is because how we think shapes what we notice when we look at the world (and ourselves).
- We tend to see and give more weight to evidence that fits or supports what we already think or believe.
- We tend to *not* notice evidence that goes against our existing thoughts, or, if we do, we often discount it, or minimize how relevant or important it is.

When might I have trauma-based thoughts?

Trauma-based thoughts typically happen when something reminds you of something emotionally overwhelming from your past.

How can I help myself notice I might be having trauma-based thoughts?

This difficult but important work is made possible by relating to your reactions with curiosity and self-compassion.

What are signs I might be having trauma-based thoughts?

Without minimizing things in the present that are not OK, get curious when:

- you are having an intense or overwhelming emotion
- a situation feels "like" or "just like" something from the past, or you feel you "have" to do something
- you are having an intensely negative reaction to someone
- you are having intensely negative thoughts about yourself.

What are the steps to manage trauma-based thoughts?

If you find yourself having a very strong emotional reaction,

1. **Get grounded/use healthy coping skills.**

   It is always easier to see things more clearly, notice and think about what is happening and your available options, and decide what is best to do when you are grounded.

2. **Get curious.**
   - Is there something I am missing?
   - Are there things I am not paying attention to?
   - Do I have strengths and resources that I'm not keeping in mind?
   - Am I being fair?

3. **Give yourself credit if you are able to notice something you had missed.**

4. **Work to change your thinking** if you notice you have been unfair to yourself or others or have inaccurately assessed the safety of a situation.

Remember:

Each time you work toward helping yourself notice trauma-based thoughts helps your brain get better at noticing when you are safer, trim fear pathways, and build new, calm, healthy pathways. **Each effort you make** (whether you notice or not!) **helps toward your goal!**

EXERCISES FOR TOPIC 11: MANAGING TRAUMA-BASED THOUGHTS

We hope you have been working to be patient and compassionate with yourself as you learn to use healthy skills. We also hope you have been reminding yourself that learning to do things differently takes time and repeated practice, and that you are giving yourself credit for each bit of progress.

In the information sheet for Topic 11, we talked about trauma-based thoughts, including how to notice them and the importance of helping you manage and change them. Please review the information sheet before continuing on to the exercises below, which focus on identifying and managing trauma-based thoughts.

As with all work in this program, we recommend making sure you are grounded before beginning this work. We also want to remind you that it is not only OK but also important to notice when you need to take a break in order to get grounded. (Taking breaks to get grounded is an example of self-compassionately giving yourself the care you need.)

The goal is for you to get and feel safer. Pausing whatever you are doing to get grounded when you notice that you are ungrounded is actually one of the most important ways you can help yourself make progress toward getting and feeling safer.

Written Exercise for Topic 11: Managing Trauma-Based Thoughts

Identifying and managing trauma-based thoughts
Trauma-based thoughts are based on beliefs that are not true (or are no longer true), but they feel true based on traumatic experiences. Trauma-based thoughts often help people stay safer in unsafe situations, and can be hard to think about, but are important to recognize. However, as true as they can seem, they are generally distorted or harsh. It is important to recognize when you are having thoughts that are not true in order to help yourself get and feel safer.

Healing from untrue and hurtful thoughts takes time. It begins with noticing that some of your thoughts may be untrue and unfair, while recognizing that there are understandable reasons why you are having such thoughts.

Please review the section of the information sheet for Topic 11 titled What Are Signs I Might Be Having Trauma-Based Thoughts? (p. 83).

Are you aware of having any trauma-based thoughts, or do you suspect that some of your thoughts might be trauma-based? If so, please list those thoughts here:

_____

_____

_____

_____

_____

_____

If you were able to notice having (or potentially having) trauma-based thoughts, try to remind yourself of this possibility when you notice yourself having those thoughts. This will help make managing them a little bit easier. (Also, note that you can get distance from trauma-based thoughts by using containment imagery to "put them away.")

If you were able to notice (or suspect) having trauma-based thoughts, is there one that feels manageable to spend a little time evaluating? If yes, please review the list of thinking mistakes that we're all at risk of making (p. 36) and continue to the next step, below.

A good starting place for managing trauma-based thoughts is to ask yourself what you would tell someone you care about if they were in the same situation. What would you tell them about how they are thinking about themselves?

(For example: Would it be fair for someone else to think this way? What would you tell them to notice when they are being too self-critical?)

_____

_____

_____

_____

_____

_____

_____

_____

When you are ready, it is helpful to look for signs or evidence that these thoughts may not be true. You can make a list of the evidence that challenges the untrue and unfair thoughts, and review that list regularly.

As you come up with challenges that you intellectually know to be true, write them down whether or not you believe them emotionally. (Said another way, you might know in your head that something is evidence against a trauma-based thought even though the thought may still feel very true in your heart.)

Things I have noticed at least once that suggest the thought is not true:

(Example: I think I cannot get better, but there have been a couple of times using these techniques that helped me feel better for a little while.)

_____

_____

_____

_____

_____

_____

_____

_____

_____

_____

_____

_____

TIP: Consider reading over the challenges to trauma-based thoughts multiple times a day, even when things are going well. Over time, you will notice more evidence against unfair, untrue, and unhelpful thoughts. You will notice experiences that help create more fair and helpful thoughts that will make it easier to get and feel safer. Add this evidence to your list of things you have noticed that suggest the trauma-based thought is not true.

Practice Exercise for Topic 11: Managing Trauma-Based Thoughts

We encourage you to continue to practice being compassionate with yourself using GIVE and CARE, especially when things are challenging.

We also encourage you to allow yourself to notice whether you might be having trauma-based thoughts. Look for evidence that suggests these thoughts are untrue or unfair. As you notice things that don't fit with or that contradict the trauma-based belief, add that evidence to your list of things you have noticed that suggest the trauma-based thought is not true. Take time to review this list regularly.

Please be patient and compassionate with yourself as you go through the process of learning to use these skills, reminding yourself that learning how to do things differently takes time and repeated practice. As you are ready, consider taking your potential trauma-based thoughts to therapy for help finding evidence that suggests the thoughts are not true or not fair.

And don't forget to notice and give yourself credit for each bit of progress—each effort you make makes a difference in helping your brain (and all of who you are) heal!

> *TIP:* As you continue through the program, strive to integrate what you've been learning into your daily routines. We recognize that this is much easier said than done, so please be patient with yourself as you work toward getting better and better at:
> - working to keep yourself grounded
> - separating the past from the present
> - giving yourself the care you need to help heal trauma's impact on the brain
> - being curious about (and challenging) potential trauma-based thoughts, and
> - noticing and giving yourself credit for progress.

Congratulations on completing the third module! Step by step, you're getting there!

In the modules that follow, we'll offer additional information and skills to help you keep making progress toward getting and feeling safer.

Getting and Feeling Safer, Part 1

This module focuses on recognizing and interrupting patterns that increase your risk of doing things that are risky, unhealthy, or unsafe, and things you can do instead to help yourself get and feel safer.

This module will help you learn:

- to recognize and plan how to manage challenging situations
- why getting healthy needs met safely is so important for your healing
- why people who have experienced trauma sometimes do unhealthy or unsafe things, and how to get healthier and safer
- the cycle of unhealthy behavior and how to break out of it
- trauma-related reactions and how to reduce them.

This module will help you practice:

- managing challenging situations
- recognizing and meeting your healthy needs
- noticing and responding to early warning signs
- breaking the cycle of unhealthy behavior
- reducing trauma-related reactions.

This difficult, important work builds on all you've already done as part of this program to help you make meaningful progress toward getting and feeling safer. Please give yourself the care you need as you do this work.

RECOGNIZING AND PLANNING HOW TO MANAGE CHALLENGING SITUATIONS

Information Sheet for Topic 12

What is not challenging for one person can be very challenging for another—and often, the reason the situation is challenging is because it reminds them of past difficult or traumatic situations. It is usually easier to notice which situations can be challenging—and what might help—after the fact. Getting curious about what might have helped in these situations can help you plan for how to respond in a way that is more likely to be helpful next time.

Triggers and how to manage them

- Difficult situations that can overwhelm your ability to cope or manage effectively are commonly referred to as "triggers."
- The term "trigger" can refer to anything that generally leads you to have difficulty coping.
- Being aware of your triggers prepares you to manage your responses to them safely.
- Although coping with triggers can be very difficult, it is possible—and gets easier with practice. The more detailed your plan for how you will cope with triggers, and the more practice you have managing them, the easier it will get.
- Be mindful of situations where you are likely to be exposed to a trigger; this will help you plan in advance for how you will manage it. If you know that you are likely to be exposed to a particular trigger, keep in mind how you will respond to it.
- Use healthy coping to manage triggers. We have talked about a number of different healthy coping techniques; encourage yourself to try and practice each of these so you will know what helps you (and how to help yourself) when you are triggered.

TIPS:

- Do not needlessly trigger yourself. Avoidance of safe situations is unhealthy; so is unnecessary exposure to highly triggering situations. Unnecessary exposure to highly triggering situations gets in the way of helping you get and feel safer.
- Strive to not expose yourself to highly triggering situations, including movies, TV shows, social media, images, and music that contain highly triggering material.

EXERCISES FOR TOPIC 12: RECOGNIZING AND PLANNING HOW TO MANAGE CHALLENGING SITUATIONS

We hope you have continued to practice giving yourself the care you need, especially when things are challenging. We also hope you have begun to allow yourself to notice and challenge trauma-based thoughts.

In the information sheet for Topic 12, we talked about planning how to manage challenging situations. Please review the information sheet before continuing on to the exercises below, which focus on identifying and managing triggers.

Written Exercises for Topic 12: Recognizing and Planning How to Manage Challenging Situations

It is easier to notice which situations are difficult for us and what we could have done to help ourselves *after* difficult situations are over. These exercises encourage you to identify situations that can be difficult for you, and to make specific plans for how to manage them.

As part of this work, we will ask you to think about past times when coping was difficult. As with all work in this program, we recommend making sure you are grounded before beginning this work, and we encourage you to take breaks to get grounded if you start to feel too much or too little. The goal is for you to get and feel safer. Put safety and healthy coping first.

(Remember: Taking breaks to get grounded as you need to is an example of self-compassionately giving yourself the care you need. Pausing whatever you are doing to help yourself get grounded is actually one of the most important ways you can help yourself make progress toward getting and feeling safer.)

This can be a challenging topic, so be sure to pace yourself, working on it a little bit at a time. Take breaks as often as you need them. We encourage you to talk to your therapist about this topic; your therapist might have good suggestions about what could help you in situations where you have difficulty remembering or using healthy coping.

Written exercise 1: Identifying your triggers
Read the questions below to help yourself identify feelings, thoughts, or situations that trigger difficulty with safety or unhealthy behaviors. These questions may help you notice different situations that trigger you.

Are there particular **Times** of day, week, month, or year that tend to trigger you?

_____

_____

_____

_____

_____

_____

Are there particular **Places** that tend to trigger you?

_____

_____

_____

_____

_____

_____

Are there particular **Situations** that tend to trigger you?
(Possible examples: Crowded places; small spaces; being alone and feeling lonely; being with someone who is angry or upset with you; being with someone saying something nice about you.)

_____

_____

_____

_____

_____

Are there particular **Emotions** that tend to trigger you?
(Possible examples: Shame, loneliness, anger, emptiness, wanting to be cared for, sadness, fear, happiness.)

_____

_____

_____

_____

_____

_____

Are there particular **Sensations** that tend to trigger you?
(Sights? Sounds? Smells? Tastes? Textures?)

_____

_____

_____

_____

_____

Are there particular **Thoughts** that tend to trigger you?
(Common examples: "I am bad," "I am damaged," "I am broken," "I'm all alone," "There's no hope,"
"No one cares," or "I want someone to care, but that's wrong and it will never happen.")

_____

_____

_____

_____

_____

_____

Written exercise 2: Managing your triggers

As you identify your triggers, it is important to identify healthy, safe ways of managing them. It may be helpful to consult past information sheets and exercises as you go through the process of identifying healthy ways to manage triggers.

You may also find the following suggestions helpful.

TIPS:

- Triggering **Times** and **Places** (and triggering **Situations** you know about ahead of time) are best managed by having a plan for what you can do before, during, and after the difficult time, place, or situation. (For guidance on how to approach this, see the "Making a Before, During, and After (BDA) Plan" worksheet on p. 97. This worksheet can help you prepare yourself to manage these times, places, and situations.) You will get even better managing triggering times, places, and situations as you gain more experience through practice.

- Triggering **Emotions** and **Sensations** can be made more bearable by orienting and anchoring, using some of the 101 Healthy Ways to Get and Stay Grounded, Separating Past from Present (including being curious about 90/10 reactions), and the imagery techniques we have talked about. Triggering **Sensations** can also be counteracted with *different* sensations (such as a pleasant sight, sound, smell, taste, or texture). For example, if you find the cold to be triggering, you could find ways to keep warm (e.g., putting on layers of clothing) and remind yourself, "I can take steps now to keep warm and take care of myself. Now is different from the past."

- If you find yourself triggered by **Thoughts**, challenge the thoughts. Ask yourself: What would I tell a good friend in a similar situation who thought these things about themselves? Write this down. Remind yourself that although it might feel like the new thought does not fit for you, it is only fair that the same statements apply to you as they would to a friend.

With all the above in mind, enter your triggers into the left-hand column of the table below, adding healthy ways to manage them in the right-hand column.

Trigger	*Healthy ways to manage/cope with trigger*

Trigger	Healthy ways to manage/cope with trigger

Practice Exercise for Topic 12: Recognizing and Planning How to Manage Challenging Situations

We encourage you to practice using healthy ways of coping with triggers. Taking action to be ready with a plan for difficult situations helps you heal. It also makes it much more likely that you will be able to help yourself interrupt the process of getting overwhelmed and cope in a healthy way.

We also encourage you to continue to practice being compassionate with yourself and giving yourself the care you need, especially when things are challenging—like when facing triggers or trauma-based thoughts.

Please be patient with yourself as you go through the process of learning to use healing-focused coping skills. Remind yourself that learning how to do things differently takes time and repeated practice.

Don't forget to notice and give yourself credit for each bit of progress—each effort you make makes a difference in helping your brain (and all of who you are) heal.

Step by step, you will get there!

ADDITIONAL RESOURCE

Making a Before, During, and After (BDA) plan

Making a plan for what to do before, during, and after a difficult situation can improve your ability to manage difficult situations.

Consider making a Before, During, and After (BDA) plan[1] for situations that you think could evoke difficult emotions, symptoms, or unhealthy impulses.

Before: The "Before" part of the plan should consist of things you can to do prepare yourself for successfully managing the event:

- What can you do that will help you be better prepared to handle the situation well?
- How far ahead of time should you begin?
- Consider including specific healthy grounding/relaxation/self-soothing skills as well as healthy self-talk. Depending on the situation, healthy self-talk may consist of:
    - reminding yourself of differences between the past and the upcoming situation (separating past from present), including reminding yourself of the strengths and resources you now have access to; and
    - giving yourself encouragement for developing a plan for what you will do during the event.

During: The "During" part of the plan should consist of things you can do to help yourself continue to be effective throughout the situation. This should include specific things you plan to do to keep yourself grounded. Depending on the situation, it may also include a script for what you want to say and do, and a list of topics to not talk about or things not to do.

After: The "After" part of the plan should consist of things you can do after the situation to help yourself self-soothe in a healthy way. This part of the plan should also include giving yourself credit for having managed the situation in a healthy way.

You may find it helpful to discuss your plan with others who you trust for feedback and/or additional ideas.

Reference for Topic 12

Trauma Disorders Program, Sheppard Pratt Health System—Patient handouts, v. 2013.

---

[1] "Before, During, and After Plan" adapted from Sheppard Pratt Trauma Disorders Unit Patient Handouts, v. 2013.

GETTING HEALTHY NEEDS MET SAFELY

Information Sheet for Topic 13

Getting healthy needs met safely keeps people doing well and makes it possible for people to heal and grow. At the same time, it is not unusual for people with trauma histories to have difficulty taking healthy care of themselves.

How does getting healthy needs met safely help heal trauma?

Over time, the more a person is able to get their healthy needs met safely:

- The less stressed/anxious they are.
- The more they are able to handle stressful and challenging situations well.
- The less likely they are to get overwhelmed by stressful and challenging situations.
- The more they begin to feel OK.

Why do people with trauma histories sometimes have difficulty taking healthy care of themselves?

There are multiple reasons why getting healthy needs met safely can be difficult for people with trauma histories; the more of these are true, the harder it can be:

- They were never shown how to take healthy care of themselves.
- They are still in the process of learning healthy ways of helping themselves.
- They are still in the process of learning how to relate to themselves with healthy self-compassion.
- Trauma-based beliefs make them think they do not deserve to be healthy and safe.

How can I get better at taking healthy care of myself?

- Practice relating to yourself with healthy self-compassion:
  - Give yourself the care you need. Relate to yourself using **GIVE CARE**.
- When you have a difficult time doing this:
  - **Get curious** if you might be struggling with trauma-based thoughts.
  - Give yourself credit if you notice you are, and work to manage these thoughts.
  - **Act "as if"**: Do what you would do if you were not having trauma-based thoughts. Consider what you would tell, recommend to, or do for a child or adult you care about in the same situation. Do the same for yourself.

EXERCISES FOR TOPIC 13: GETTING HEALTHY NEEDS MET SAFELY

We hope you have been practicing using healthy ways of coping with triggers, and being compassionate with yourself, especially when things are challenging—like when facing triggers or trauma-based thoughts.

In the information sheet for Topic 13, we talked about "Getting Healthy Needs Met Safely." Please review this information before continuing on to the exercises below, which focus on helping make this process more understandable.

Written Exercises for Topic 13: Getting Healthy Needs Met Safely

Written exercise 1: Identifying how often you are able to get your healthy needs met safely
In the information sheet for Topic 13, we talked about how getting healthy needs met safely keeps people doing well and makes it possible to heal and grow. One of the reasons that people who have experienced trauma can have difficulty taking care of themselves is that trauma can lead people to believe their needs are not OK. With this in mind, this exercise offers a list of healthy needs and encourages you to consider whether you are currently getting these needs met safely.

As with all work in this program, we recommend making sure you are grounded before beginning this work. Take breaks to get grounded when you start to feel too much or too little. Our goal is for you to get and feel safer. Please put safety and healthy coping first.

This can be a challenging topic, so be sure to pace yourself, taking breaks as often as you need them. We also encourage you to talk to your therapist about how to get more of your healthy needs met in safe and healthy ways.

Are you grounded?

Please review the list of healthy needs below. For each, rate the degree you are getting that healthy need met safely by circling the percentage of time you are able to meet that healthy need.

How often are you able to get these healthy needs met safely?

Shelter *(a physically and emotionally safe place to live)*

0%	10	20	30	40	50	60	70	80	90	100%
(never)										(always)

Sustenance *(healthy food to eat)*

0%	10	20	30	40	50	60	70	80	90	100%
(never)										(always)

Rest *(healthy sleep, relaxation)*

0%	10	20	30	40	50	60	70	80	90	100%
(never)										(always)

Connection/Belonging *(safe and healthy relationships)*

0%	10	20	30	40	50	60	70	80	90	100%
(never)										(always)

Recreation *(healthy activities that you find relaxing, invigorating, or fun)*

0%	10	20	30	40	50	60	70	80	90	100%
(never)										(always)

Meaningful Activity *(healthy activities that you find inherently meaningful)*

0%	10	20	30	40	50	60	70	80	90	100%
(never)										(always)

Remember:

Over time, the more a person is able to get their healthy needs met safely:

- The less stressed/anxious they are
- The more they are able to handle stressful and challenging situations well
- The less likely they are to get overwhelmed by stressful and challenging situations
- The more they begin to feel OK.

Working to get your healthy needs met safely is a powerful way to help you get and feel safer.

Written exercise 2: Getting more of your healthy needs met safely

In Written Exercise 1, you considered how often you are getting your healthy needs met safely. Review your answers for Shelter, Sustenance, Rest, Connection/Belonging, Recreation, and Meaningful Activity. Use the space below to identify manageable changes you can make that would help you get more of your healthy needs met safely.

(Remember, each bit of progress you make toward getting more of your healthy needs met safely helps!)

_____

_____

_____

_____

_____

_____

_____

_____

_____

_____

_____

_____

_____

_____

Written exercise 3: What to avoid doing: Trying to meet healthy needs in unealthy ways
Written Exercises 1 and 2 encouraged you to work toward getting your healthy needs met safely. Unfortunately, it is common for people to try to get their healthy needs (Shelter, Sustenance, Rest, Connection/Belonging, Recreation, and Meaningful Activity) met in unhealthy ways. (We'll be talking about the many reasons why this can be true in the next topic.)

The table below describes three of the most common unhealthy ways that people try to get their healthy needs met, why to avoid them, and what you can do instead. Please review the table and consider how this information might be helpful for you.

What to avoid	Why to avoid it	What to do instead
Isolating Avoiding being around safe people; staying alone, not communicating with, and/or not responding to, safe people	Avoiding being around safe people keeps you from having healthy connections and feelings of belonging. Isolating can also lead to thinking more about upsetting thoughts or feelings, which can increase depression and unsafe impulses.	*Do the opposite:* Rather than isolate, encourage yourself to spend time with safe people. Spend time in safe public places. Stay in communication with safe people. Reach out to safe people to do healthy, fun things, or for distraction. Talk to treatment providers if you have difficulty with safety or risky/unhealthy behaviors. *Underlying need to meet in healthy ways:* • *Connection/Belonging* (*if isolating because of not trusting people who are safe or because of feeling shame*)
Self-medicating Drinking alcohol, using illegal drugs, or misusing prescription medications to help yourself manage difficult emotions/ situations	When people use drugs or drink alcohol, their judgment worsens, and their thinking becomes less rational. They are more likely to engage in risky, unhealthy, or unsafe behavior.	Use healthy, recovery-focused skills to help yourself when feeling too much or too little, like the skills described in this program. If you are self-medicating, please talk about these problems with your therapist, and work toward identifying healthy ways to get your underlying needs (see below) met safely. If you continue to have difficulty reducing self-medicating, consider attending an appropriate recovery group. It can be very difficult, if not impossible, to get over these problems alone. Recovery groups are very useful for many people. In many places, there are 12-step recovery groups such as Alcoholics Anonymous or Narcotics Anonymous. Find resources near you. *Underlying needs to meet in healthy ways:* • *Rest* (*if wanting to feel relaxed*) • *Recreation* (*if wanting to have fun*) • *Connection/Belonging* (*if using alcohol/drugs to connect with others*)

What to avoid	Why to avoid it	What to do instead
Ruminating Repeatedly thinking about hurtful, critical, or unfair thoughts or messages, especially messages from people who hurt you or did not take good care of you	It can be very difficult to stop believing hurtful messages from others, especially those from childhood. Children are vulnerable to believing what they are told. If people said painful things to you in childhood, those messages probably made you feel awful about yourself. Repeating those things to yourself now, as an adult, is likely to make you feel bad about yourself now.	Be compassionate with yourself; give yourself the care you need using GIVE CARE. Remind yourself that false beliefs about being a bad person are very common among people who experienced trauma. These old messages can make people depressed and self-destructive. Instead of ruminating on them, allow yourself to practice letting them go. When you start thinking about old hurtful messages, it might be helpful to say, "That is what I heard long ago, but it is not true." (Or maybe as a first step, "It is not necessarily true all the time.") "The person who told me that didn't know how to treat children in healthy ways." Or use imagery: Think about letting thoughts go like you would let a balloon float up and away in the sky. Some of you might have parts or voices that repeat painful messages. If that is true, you might try asking the part/voice if they could please not be so harsh. Could they try easing up on those old messages? ***Underlying need to meet in healthy ways:*** • ***Connection/Belonging*** *(the example described reviewing hurtful messages from people; our minds typically do this to try to understand why we did not have healthy relationships with important people in our lives)*

TIP: Isolating, self-medicating, and ruminating interfere with experiences that can help you feel better

- *Isolating* keeps you from being able to have experiences where nothing bad (or something good) happens.
- *Self-medicating* keeps you from feeling the feelings that are telling you something may *not* be OK, and can make it harder to notice things that *are* OK. (Using drugs and alcohol or misusing prescriptions can have many other negative effects, too.)
- *Ruminating* can keep you from noticing positive things that do not fit with old, critical thoughts.

Do you engage in isolating, self-medicating, or ruminating?

If yes, please use this space to describe what you will do to help change these patterns into healthier ways of getting your needs met:

_____

_____

_____

_____

_____

_____

_____

_____

_____

_____

Written exercise 4: Finding starting points for getting safer

Knowing what safety feels like may help you know what you can accomplish by working toward getting and feeling safer.

For some people, safety feels like being comfortable.

Think about safe (or safer) situations when you have felt at least some degree of comfort. Can you remember what your body felt like? *(For example, were your shoulders tense, or relaxed?)* Can you remember your emotions? *(Did you feel anxious, or relatively calm and happy?)*

Write about what you feel like when you are in safe (or safer) situations where you feel at least somewhat comfortable, peaceful, and/or relaxed. Include descriptions of what you notice about your mood, your thoughts, and how your body feels in these situations.

_____

_____

_____

_____

_____

_____

_____

_____

_____

_____

For other people, safety means feeling OK in the world and/or OK with yourself and others. Think about situations where you have felt more OK in the world, more OK with yourself, or more OK in your relationships with other people. Please describe what these experiences are like.

(What do you notice in your body? What do you notice about your mood or your thoughts about yourself?)

_____

_____

_____

_____

_____

_____

_____

_____

_____

_____

_____

_____

_____

_____

Practice Exercise for Topic 13: Getting Healthy Needs Met Safely

We encourage you to see if you can begin to work toward getting your healthy needs met more safely. We also encourage you to continue to practice being compassionate with yourself and giving yourself the care you need, especially when things are challenging—like when facing triggers or trauma-based thoughts.

Please be patient with yourself as you go through the process of learning to use healing-focused coping skills, reminding yourself that learning how to do things differently takes time and repeated practice.

Don't forget to notice and give yourself credit for each bit of progress—each step you take makes a difference in helping your brain (and all of who you are) heal!

Step by step, you will get there!

WHY PEOPLE WHO HAVE EXPERIENCED TRAUMA SOMETIMES DO RISKY, UNHEALTHY, OR UNSAFE THINGS, AND HOW TO GET HEALTHIER AND SAFER

Information Sheet for Topic 14

Getting healthy needs met safely keeps people doing well and makes it possible for people to heal and grow. Unfortunately, many people with trauma histories want to get and feel safer *and* have difficulty taking healthy care of themselves.

Why do people with trauma histories sometimes do risky, unhealthy, or unsafe things?[2]

There are multiple factors that can lead people to do these kinds of things. Reasons that may play a role include:

- Because they were never shown how to take healthy care of themselves.
- Because these things seem to help them feel better *(in the short term)*:
  - to distract from difficult feelings/change the way they feel,
  - to feel more in control, and/or
  - to feel less overwhelmed or dissociated.
- Because they are still in the process of learning healthy ways to help themselves when feeling too much or too little.
- Because they do not yet trust that healthy ways can really help.
- Because they are still in the process of learning how to relate to themselves with healthy self-compassion.
- Because trauma-based beliefs make them think they do not deserve to be healthy and safe.
- If they hear voices, to temporarily quiet voices, or to get voices to be less critical.
- Because these things help them not act on even more risky, unhealthy, or dangerous impulses.

---

[2] Informed in part by a list by Boon et al., 2011, p. 316.

How do these behaviors get in the way of healing from trauma?

While these behaviors can seem to help in the short term, they:

- contribute to feeling unsafe,
- interfere with making progress toward healing and recovery, and
- implicitly reinforce the idea that you do not deserve to be safe and healthy.

To get and feel safer, please work to get your healthy needs met safely.

How do these behaviors keep people stuck in a cycle of feeling unsafe?

Repeated unhealthy, risky, and/or unsafe behaviors lead people to be stuck in a cycle of mistreating themselves and feeling bad because:

- These behaviors do not fix the underlying problem(s).
- They only "work" for a short time.
- The feelings/problems come back.
- When the underlying problems come back, they are often bigger than before.
- When the behaviors relate to past traumas, they keep a person stuck in a pattern of retraumatizing themselves and/or reliving aspects of an unsafe past.
- They keep a person stuck with feelings from the past without therapeutically addressing them and helping the person gradually get freer from them.
- It means that the person is missing opportunities to practice and get better at using healthy ways of managing trauma-related reactions and powerful emotions.
- These behaviors send a message to the person that it is OK to be at risk, unhealthy, unsafe, hurt, or not cared for—a message that is not true and not OK.

How can I help myself get healthier and safer?

- Give yourself the care you need. Strive toward taking healthy care of yourself, and getting your healthy needs met safely. The more you are able to do this, the easier it will be to change these kinds of behaviors.

- Work to notice:
  - which situations tend to trigger or put you at risk for these behaviors,
  - "warning signs" that you might be at risk for these behaviors, and develop plans for how to help yourself with recovery-focused coping skills, like the ones in this program.
- If you find yourself having strong emotions, or have difficulty giving yourself the care you need:
  - **Get curious** if you might be struggling with trauma-based thoughts.
  - **Give yourself credit** if you notice you are, **and work to manage these thoughts**.
  - **Act "as if"**: Do what you would do if you were not having trauma-based thoughts. Consider what you would tell, recommend to, or do for a child or adult you care about in the same situation. Do the same for yourself.
- **Approach this work with healthy self-compassion:** Changing how you do things takes lots of practice over time. Step by step, you'll get there!

EXERCISES FOR TOPIC 14: WHY PEOPLE WHO HAVE EXPERIENCED TRAUMA SOMETIMES DO RISKY, UNHEALTHY, OR UNSAFE THINGS, AND HOW TO GET HEALTHIER AND SAFER

We hope you have been working toward getting your healthy needs met more safely, and have been practicing being compassionate with yourself, especially when things are challenging—like when facing triggers or trauma-based thoughts.

In the information sheet for Topic 14, we talked about why people who have experienced trauma sometimes do risky, unhealthy, or unsafe things; how these behaviors get in the way of healing from trauma; and how to get healthier and safer. Please review this information before continuing on to the exercises below, which focus on helping you identify warning signs that suggest you might be at risk for doing something risky, unhealthy, or unsafe.

Written Exercises for Topic 14: Why People Who Have Experienced Trauma Sometimes Do Risky, Unhealthy, or Unsafe Things, and How to Get Healthier and Safer

In the information sheet for Topic 14, we recommended working to notice warning signs that you might be at risk for doing risky, unhealthy, or unsafe things and to develop plans to instead help yourself with healing-focused coping skills. This exercise will guide you through that process.

This can be a challenging topic, so be sure to do this at a pace that is manageable for you, taking breaks as often as you need them. As with all work in this program, we recommend making sure you are grounded before beginning this work and taking breaks to ground if you start to feel too much or too little. Our goal is for you to get and feel safer—please put safety and healthy coping first.

We also encourage you to talk to your therapist about this subject.

Are you grounded?

Once you are, think about what thoughts, emotions, physical sensations, and behaviors tend to happen before you have difficulty managing unsafe impulses, and list them under the prompts that follow.

Written exercise 1: Identifying your early warning signs

Are there particular **Thoughts** you tend to have before having a difficult time managing impulses to do something risky, unhealthy, or unsafe?

_____

_____

_____

_____

_____

_____

_____

_____

Are there particular **Emotions** you tend to have before having a difficult time managing impulses to do something risky, unhealthy, or unsafe?

(Possible examples: Shame, loneliness, anger, emptiness, wanting to be cared for, sadness, fear, happiness.)

_____

_____

_____

_____

_____

Are there particular **Physical Sensations** you tend to have before having a difficult time managing impulses to do something risky, unhealthy, or unsafe?

_____

_____

_____

_____

_____

Are there particular **Behaviors** you tend to do before having a difficult time managing impulses to do something risky, unhealthy, or unsafe?

_____

_____

_____

_____

_____

_____

_____

_____

Written exercise 2: Responding to early warning signs
Are you doing OK? Do you need a break to get grounded and practice healthy coping? If so, please do, and then come back.

Ready to continue? Let's think about ways to help you when you notice your early warning signs. One way of doing this is by creating a warning signs safety plan[3] that lists what you will do when you become aware of experiencing warning signs.

Warning signs safety plan example

Warning signs	Safety plan
Earliest warning signs: • I feel like I'm a bad or weak person. • I'm avoiding leaving the house.	**I will help myself use healthy coping by:** 1. Reviewing a list of things I tend to forget in these situations. Examples: "I'm trying to heal even though it's hard." "These warning signs are alarm signals that give me information that I need to take care of myself. They are *not* signs of weakness or failure. I can be wise and listen to these signs so I don't fall into the same old behaviors and feel ashamed." 2. Instead of isolating and getting stuck in negative thinking, I'll do something that helps me feel the opposite. Examples: I'll go for a walk outdoors, take my dog to the park, listen to uplifting music.

---

[3] Reprinted with permission of Guilford Press. Handout 2, "Create a Safety Plan" Najavits, 2002, pg. 196. [Najavits, L. M. (2002). Seeking safety: A treatment manual for PTSD and substance abuse. New York: The Guilford Press.]

Warning signs	Safety plan
I'm at increased risk when: I'm beginning to think about "quick fixes" (something risky, unhealthy, or unsafe that seems to help me feel better for a little bit).	**I will help myself use healthy coping by:** 1. Reminding myself that the old ways don't help in the long run and they make me feel more and more hopeless if I give in to them. 2. Doing something safe to feel good. Example: Going to a coffee shop to be around people and treating myself to a nice cup of coffee or tea. 3. Reaching out to someone who is supportive.
It's an emergency when: I'm getting materials together to hurt myself.	**I will stay safe by:** 1. Calling my therapist. 2. Calling a suicide hotline. 3. Going to the hospital.

Making your own warning signs safety plan

Use the table below to help you plan healthy, safe ways of responding to your warning signs. Most people find it helpful if they are very specific about the behaviors they will do when they are having trouble. We tend not to think clearly or remember well when we are upset, so it is helpful to write specific, concrete things you can do when you get into difficulty.

For example, rather than writing, "Remember one good thing about myself," actually write down a few of those good things about yourself so you can read them when you are too upset to think clearly.

It may be helpful to consult past information sheets and exercises as you go through the process of creating your own warning signs safety plan.

Warning signs safety plan

Warning signs	Safety plan
Earliest warning signs: 1. 2. 3. 4. 5.	**I will help myself use healthy coping by:** 1. 2. 3. 4. 5.
I'm at increased risk when: 1. 2. 3. 4. 5.	**I will help myself use healthy coping by:** 1. 2. 3. 4. 5.
It's an emergency when: 1. 2. 3. 4. 5.	**I will stay safe by:** 1. 2. 3. 4. 5.

Practice Exercise for Topic 14: Why People Who Have Experienced Trauma Sometimes Do Risky, Unhealthy, or Unsafe Things, and How to Get Healthier and Safer

We encourage you to be on the lookout for your early warning signs so you can be ready to practice healthy coping (using the things you listed in the "safety plan" column) as early as possible. You may find it helpful to use the early warning signs check-sheet in the Additional Resources (see p. 117) to remind you to look out for early warning signs and record the skills you used.

> *Remember:* Taking action in response to your early warning signs makes it much more likely you will be able to avoid getting overwhelmed; it also makes it much easier to cope in a healthy way.

We also encourage you to continue to practice getting your healthy needs met safely and being compassionate with yourself, especially when things are challenging—like when facing trauma-based thoughts, triggers, and warning signs.

Don't forget to notice and give yourself credit for each bit of progress—each step you take makes a difference in helping your brain (and all of who you are) heal! Be compassionate with yourself as you practice—step by step, you will get there!

ADDITIONAL RESOURCES

Understanding and preventing behaviors you want to change[4]

Follow the steps described below to better understand choices you have made and how to do things differently in the future. As always, pause to work on getting grounded if you start to feel too much or too little.

1. **Describe the problem** (e.g., risky, unhealthy, or unsafe behavior) you are trying to understand and prevent **at a headline level** (i.e., in the way a newspaper would summarize the behavior you'd like to change in a headline).
2. **Describe what happened before you did the thing you are trying to change.** Questions that may help you with this:
   A. What was **happening** before the problem started?
   B. What were you **thinking, feeling, imagining,** or **doing?**

---

[4] Reprinted with permission of Guilford Press. General Handout 7a, pg. 21-22. Linehan, M. (2015), DBT skills training handouts and worksheets, second edition. New York: The Guilford Press.

    C.   What was **different** about this situation than other situations where the problem does not happen?

3. **Vulnerability factors:** There are a number of things that make us more vulnerable to/ likely to have problems. Were any of the following true before the problem?

    A.   Were you getting too little or too much sleep?

    B.   Were you sick? Physically ill? Physically injured?

    C.   Had you been eating too much or too little?

    D.   Had you been using substances?

    E.   Had you been drinking alcohol?

    F.   Had you been not taking prescription drugs as prescribed (e.g., missing doses or taking more than prescribed)?

    G.   Were you facing stressful situations?

    H.   Were you having strong emotions or feeling too much?

    I.   Were you feeling too little or starting to dissociate?

4. Describe the **chain of events** that led up to the problem. Imagine that the external events and your thoughts, feelings, and actions before the problem behavior (see step 2) are part of a linked chain that led up to the behavior. Ask yourself:

    A.   What happened first? Next? And after that? And after that? And after that? (Etc., etc.)

    B.   Review each link in the chain.

    C.   Ask yourself if you can break any links into smaller links.

    D.   Ask yourself which links were the earliest signs you were headed for trouble (**early warning signs**).

5. What were the short-term and longer-term **consequences** of the problem behavior?

    A.   How did *others* react to your behavior? (Immediately? Later?)

    B.   How did *you* feel after the behavior? (Immediately? Later?)

    C.   What were the *negative effects* of the problem behavior? (On you? On your relationships?)

6. **Alternate solutions:** Describe things you could do differently in response to the kinds of events that happened before the problem behavior that could have led to better results.

    A.   Go back to the chain of events.

    B.   Circle each link where you could have avoided the problem behavior if you had done something different.

    C.   What healthy coping skills could you have used at each link to avoid the problem behavior?

7. Create a detailed **prevention plan** (e.g., a **warning signs safety plan**) for how to help yourself be less vulnerable to doing the problem behavior in the future.

Early warning signs check-sheet[5]

This check-sheet can help you notice early warning signs and the need to use healthy coping. It may also help you notice what was happening that might have led to early warning signs, and which coping skills were helpful.

Please use the "Situation, early warning signs?" column to briefly describe the situation. Use the "Coping skills used" column to note what you did to help yourself safely address or manage the situation.

	Situation, early warning signs?	*Coping skills used*
7:00 AM		
7:15 AM		
7:30 AM		
7:45 AM		
8:00 AM		
8:15 AM		
8:30 AM		
8:45 AM		
9:00 AM		
9:15 AM		
9:30 AM		
9:45 AM		
10:00 AM		
10:15 AM		
10:30 AM		

---

[5] Adapted from Sheppard Pratt Patient handouts, v. 2013.

	Situation, early warning signs?	Coping skills used
10:45 AM		
11:00 AM		
11:15 AM		
11:30 AM		
11:45 AM		
12:00 PM		
12:15 PM		
12:30 PM		
12:45 PM		
1:00 PM		
1:15 PM		
1:30 PM		
1:45 PM		
2:00 PM		
2:15 PM		
2:30 PM		
2:45 PM		
3:00 PM		
3:15 PM		
3:30 PM		
3:45 PM		
4:00 PM		
4:15 PM		

	Situation, early warning signs?	Coping skills used
4:30 PM		
5:00 PM		
5:15 PM		
5:30 PM		
5:45 PM		
6:00 PM		
6:15 PM		
6:30 PM		
6:45 PM		
7:00 PM		
7:15 PM		
7:30 PM		
7:45 PM		
8:00 PM		
8:15 PM		
8:30 PM		
8:45 PM		
9:00 PM		
9:15 PM		
9:30 PM		
9:45 PM		
10:00 PM		
10:15 PM		

	Situation, early warning signs?	*Coping skills used*
10:30 PM		
10:45 PM		
11:00 PM		
11:30 PM		

References for Topic 14

Boon, S., Steele, K., & van der Hart, O. (2011). *Coping with trauma-related dissociation: Skills training for patients.* W. W. Norton & Company.

Linehan, M. (2015). *DBT skills training handouts and worksheets* (2nd ed.). Guilford Press.

Najavits, L. M. (2002). *Seeking safety: A treatment manual for PTSD and substance abuse.* Guilford Press.

Trauma Disorders Program, Sheppard Pratt Health System—Patient handouts, v. 2013.

THE CYCLE OF UNHEALTHY BEHAVIOR AND HOW TO BREAK OUT OF IT

Information Sheet for Topic 15

Many people with trauma histories end up using unhealthy behaviors to get through times when they are feeling too much or too little. Unfortunately, while these behaviors may help them feel better in the short term, they actually keep them stuck in a cycle of feeling too much or too little, unhealthy behavior, and feeling unsafe, getting in the way of healing and recovery.

How do I interrupt my cycle of unhealthy behavior?

Understanding your own cycle of unhealthy behavior is an important step toward helping you interrupt it. The cycle of unhealthy behavior[6] can be thought of as having four parts:

- *Warning signs:* The situations, physical sensations, emotions, thoughts, and behaviors that tend to happen before you have difficulty managing unhealthy impulses.
- *The last straw:* The event that you experience as breaking your ability to maintain safety. It triggers a desire to give in to urges to do unhealthy things.
- *Unhealthy behavior:* This includes any activities that put physical safety or health at risk, including self-neglect; self-medication with overeating or overuse of drugs, alcohol, or prescribed medications; risky, impulsive, and/or addictive behaviors; self-harm; suicide attempts; and aggression toward others.
- *Results:* This part includes both the short-term (or immediate) results (which usually involve some sense of relief) and the delayed (or longer-term) results of these behaviors (retriggering reactions and feelings that restart the cycle).

To interrupt a cycle of unhealthy behavior, work to replace unhealthy behaviors with healing-focused coping skills like the ones described in this program.

---

[6] Adapted from the "Cycle of Self-Harm" in Boon et al., 2011, p. 318. "Last Straw" concept: Lewis et al., 2004.

How do these behaviors get in the way of healing from trauma?

While these behaviors can seem to help in the short term, they:

- contribute to feeling unsafe, which leads to feeling too much/too little,

- interfere with making progress toward healing and recovery, and

- implicitly reinforce the idea that you do not deserve to be safe and healthy.

To get and feel safer, please work to get your healthy needs met safely.

How do these behaviors keep people stuck in a cycle of feeling unsafe?

Repeated unhealthy, risky, and/or unsafe behaviors lead people to be stuck in a cycle of mistreating themselves and feeling bad because:

- The behaviors do not fix the underlying problem(s).

- They only "work" for a short time.

- The feelings/problems come back.

- When the underlying problems come back, they are often bigger than before.

- When the behaviors relate to past traumas, they keep a person stuck in a pattern of retraumatizing themselves and/or reliving aspects of an unsafe past.

- They keep a person stuck with feelings from the past without therapeutically addressing them and helping the person gradually get freer from them.

- It means that the person is missing opportunities to practice and get better at using healthy ways of managing trauma-related reactions and powerful emotions.

- It sends a message to the person that it is OK to be at risk, unhealthy, unsafe, hurt, or not cared for—a message that is not true and not OK.

How can I help myself get healthier and safer?

Give yourself the care you need. Strive toward taking healthy care of yourself and getting your healthy needs met safely. The more you are able to do this, the easier it will be to change these kinds of behaviors.

- Work to notice:

  - which situations tend to trigger or put you at risk for these behaviors, and

  - warning signs that you might be at risk for these behaviors.

- Develop plans for how to help yourself with recovery-focused coping skills, like the ones in this program.
- If you find yourself having strong emotions, or have difficulty giving yourself the care you need:
  - **Get curious** if you might be struggling with trauma-based thoughts.
  - **Give yourself credit** if you notice you are, **and work to manage these thoughts**.
  - **Act "as if":** Do what you would do if you were not having trauma-based thoughts. Consider what you would tell, recommend to, or do for a child or adult you care about in the same situation. Do the same for yourself.
- **Approach this work with healthy self-compassion:** Changing how you do things takes lots of practice over time. Step by step, you'll get there!

EXERCISES FOR TOPIC 15: THE CYCLE OF UNHEALTHY BEHAVIOR AND HOW TO BREAK OUT OF IT

We hope you have been watching for early warning signs and practicing healthy coping early when you notice warning signs. We also hope you have been continuing to practice getting your healthy needs met more safely and are being compassionate with yourself, especially when things are challenging—like when facing trauma-based thoughts, triggers, and warning signs.

In the information sheet for Topic 15, we talked about why people who have experienced trauma often get caught in a cycle of risky, unhealthy, or unsafe behavior that keeps people stuck; how these behaviors get in the way of healing from trauma; and how to get healthier and safer. Please review this information before continuing on to the exercises below, which focus on helping identify and interrupt cycles of risky, unhealthy, and unsafe behaviors.

Written Exercises for Topic 15: The Cycle of Unhealthy Behavior and How to Break Out of It

In the information sheet for Topic 15, we emphasized that understanding your own cycle of unhealthy behavior is an important step toward helping you interrupt it. This exercise will guide you through that process. We also encourage you to talk to your therapist about this subject.

As with all work in this program, we recommend making sure you are grounded before beginning this work, and taking breaks to ground if you start to feel too much or too little. Our goal is for you to get and feel safer—please put safety and healthy coping first.

As you work on this difficult subject, please try to be compassionate with yourself. If you find yourself beginning to get critical, ask yourself: What would I tell someone I care deeply about if they were going through this exact same situation? If it is true for them, it is only fair that it is true for you, too.

Written exercise 1: Identifying and interrupting a cycle of unhealthy behavior (and an example)

Are you grounded? If yes, let's start by reviewing the cycle of unhealthy behavior and an example of a cycle of feeling too much or too little, using unhealthy behavior to try to get some sense of relief, and then feeling overwhelmed and unsafe again.

The cycle of unhealthy behavior

- *Warning signs:* The situations, physical sensations, emotions, thoughts, and behaviors that tend to happen before you have difficulty managing unhealthy impulses.
- *The last straw:* The event that you experience as breaking your ability to maintain safety. It triggers a desire to give in to urges to do unhealthy things.

- *Unhealthy behavior:* This includes any activities that put physical safety or health at risk, including self-neglect; self-medication with overeating or overuse of drugs, alcohol, or prescribed medications; risky, impulsive, and/or addictive behaviors; self-harm; suicide attempts; and aggression toward others.
- *Results:* This part includes both the short-term (or immediate) results (which usually involves some sense of relief) and the delayed (or longer-term) results of these behaviors (retriggering reactions and feelings that restart the cycle).

The cycle of unhealthy behavior: Example

- *Warning signs:* The person was isolating, having intrusive thoughts about trauma, thinking "no one likes me," and feeling unloved and lonely.
- *The last straw:* The person had an upsetting call with a friend that triggered old, unfair self-hatred and critical self-talk.
- *Unhealthy behavior:* The person started drinking, then engaged in self-harm.
- *Results:*
  - *In the short term:* The person felt some relief from painful emotions for a while.
  - *In the longer term:* The person felt ashamed. Their friends and therapist were upset. The person began to get mad at and disappointed in themselves, and began to want to withdraw and isolate, warning signs that they were at risk of restarting the cycle.

Paying attention to the longer-term results of giving in to urges to do unhealthy things is particularly important. These results include difficult feelings like self-hatred and shame that can happen after doing unhealthy things. These feelings can lead to warning signs that a person is at greater risk for doing something that feels good in the short term but puts their emotional, physical, and/or relational health at risk.

In other words, the long-term result of giving in to unhealthy behaviors is *perpetuating* unhealthy behavior.

In this example, it is easy to see how the longer-term results of unhealthy behavior are putting the person at risk for repeating the cycle: They find themselves feeling ashamed, feeling bad about themselves, and wanting to isolate again—a situation that preceded the last round of unhealthy behavior.

The shorter-term results of unhealthy behavior are temporary relief. This also puts the person at risk for repeating the cycle: Because the unhealthy behavior briefly seemed to give the person some relief, it reinforced the idea that unhealthy behavior helps, which is likely to make it harder to stop the cycle.

OK, let's think about ways the person could have interrupted the cycle. Review Figure 4.1: The Cycle of Unhealthy Behavior.[7]

---

[7] Adapted from the "Cycle of Self-Harm" in Boon et al., 2011, p. 318. "Last Straw" concept: Lewis et al., 2004.

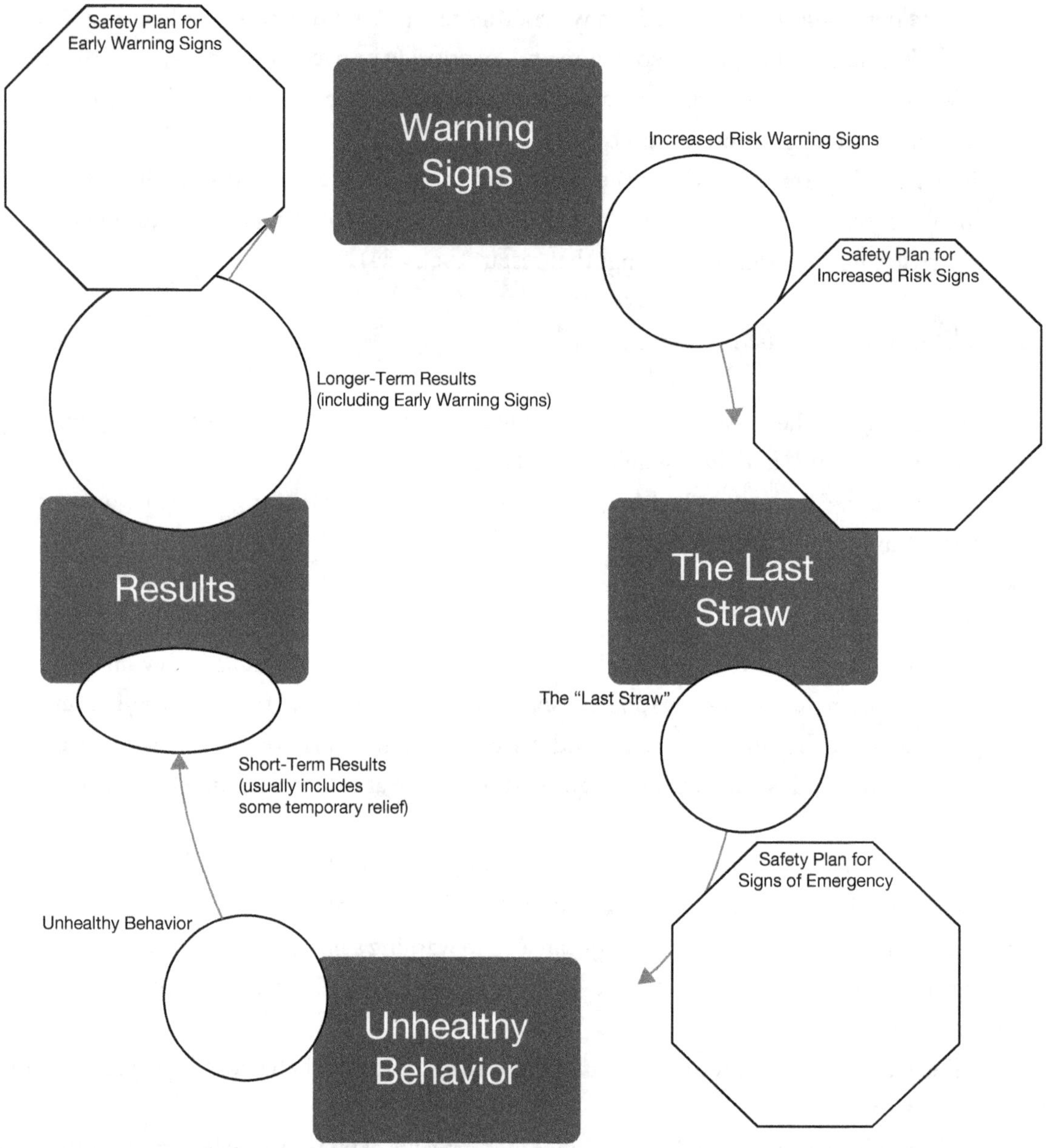

Safety Plan for
Early Warning Signs

Warning
Signs

Increased Risk Warning Signs

Safety Plan for
Increased Risk Signs

Longer-Term Results
(including Early Warning Signs)

Results

The Last
Straw

The "Last Straw"

Short-Term Results
(usually includes
some temporary relief)

Safety Plan for
Signs of Emergency

Unhealthy Behavior

Unhealthy
Behavior

FIGURE 4.1. **The Cycle of Unhealthy Behavior**

Let's think about things the person could have done at the three safety plan "action points" ("stop sign" shapes) to interrupt the cycle. What could the person do as a safety plan at the "early warning signs" point to get out of the cycle? What could the person do at the "increased risk warning signs" point to get out of the cycle? What could they do after "the last straw" but before engaging in "unhealthy behavior"?

See if you can think of things that could help at each of these points based on what you have been learning in this program: We have made space for you to write your answers in the prompts and spaces on the next page. (Feel free to look at previous information sheets and exercises while doing this!)

What could the person do as a safety plan at the "early warning signs" point (at "longer-term results," before "increased risk warning signs") to interrupt the cycle?

_____

_____

_____

_____

_____

What could the person do as a safety plan at the "increased risk warning signs" point (before "the last straw") to interrupt the cycle?

_____

_____

_____

_____

_____

What could the person do as a safety plan at the "signs of emergency" point (after "the last straw" and before "unhealthy behavior") to interrupt the cycle?

_____

_____

_____

_____

_____

Written exercise 2: Interrupting your own cycle(s) of unhealthy behavior
How are you doing? Do you need a break? If yes, please take one. When you are grounded and ready, we invite you to use Figure 4.1: The Cycle of Unhealthy Behavior to reflect on whether you might be in one or more cycles of unhealthy behavior. (Tip: Reviewing your work in the exercises for Topic 14: Why People Who Have Experienced Trauma Sometimes Do Risky, Unhealthy, or Unsafe Things, and How to Get Healthier and Safer, may help you with this.)

Remember: As always, do this work at a pace that is manageable for you. Our goal is for you to get and feel safer—please put safety and healthy coping first. Pay attention to any early warning signs that might emerge and follow your safety planning. If you start to feel overwhelmed or begin to dissociate, take a break, work on getting grounded, and practice healing-focused coping skills (things from your list of healthy things to do when feeling too much or too little).

Change takes time. You cannot and do not have to be perfect right away. Keep working at this.

TIP: If you find yourself having difficulty understanding or describing your cycle, the information on "Understanding and preventing behaviors you want to change" (pp. 115–117) can help you examine a specific incident of unhealthy behavior.

Written exercise 3: Interrupting cycles of unhealthy behavior with healthy coping cards
When you are grounded and ready, develop "healthy coping cards"[8] to help you interrupt any cycles of unhealthy behavior you have.

Using healthy coping cards can help you move from old, unsafe ways of trying to help yourself deal with triggers toward using safe, healthy ways to help yourself manage these same situations.

Healthy coping card example

Situation	How I used to respond	Safe, healthy ways to help myself
Voices in my head started getting critical of me and urging me to be unsafe. I felt self-hatred.	I felt worse and worse about myself. I told myself that maybe the voices are right, and that it might get them to be quiet if I gave in and hurt myself. Maybe then I would get some relief for a while.	I will remember that this situation is a trigger. I will remind myself that if I don't do something different, I may slip into self-harm, and then I might hate myself even more. I commit to being around other people if the voices get really critical. I will use grounding and seek distraction by doing things from the "101 Ways to Get Grounded" list. I will remind myself that these kinds of changes take a long time and that I've endured a lot worse things in my life than these feelings. I will remind myself that I can outlast these feelings.

---

[8]   Reprinted with permission of Guilford Press. Handout 4, "Safe Coping Sheet" Najavits, 2002, pg. 58. Najavits, L. M. (2002). *Seeking safety: A treatment manual for PTSD and substance abuse.* New York: The Guilford Press.

A "healthy coping results card" can help you notice the difference between what happened when you used the old way of responding versus how things go when you use a healthy, recovery-focused way to help yourself.

Healthy coping results card example

	Results of responding in the old, unsafe/unhealthy way	Results of responding in the new, healthy way
Short-term results	If I gave in, I'd feel better in the short term.	It was really hard not to use the old, unhealthy ways of coping, but eventually the feeling of needing to hurt myself decreased and I stayed safe. I was surprised and relieved.
Longer-term results	I feel like I'm not making any progress. Maybe I'm even getting worse. I feel like things will never get better, and that I don't deserve to feel better.	I'm not sure I want to fully believe it yet, but I feel like it might actually be possible for things to be different!

Use the templates below to develop your own healthy coping cards.

How to use the templates

1. Describe the situation that has most often led to you doing something risky, unhealthy, or unsafe in some way in the last few months.
   (If you find yourself wanting to use this for more than one situation, remember that you can always do more later and/or talk to your therapist about these situations. You might work on this on different days this week so that you are pacing yourself.)
2. After listing the situation, begin by writing briefly about the old ways you responded to this situation ("How I used to respond"). Then write about the short-term and longer-term effects of the old way of responding in the appropriate columns (see above for examples).

   As you complete the "longer-term results" sections for unhealthy and/or unsafe behaviors ("How I used to respond"), you might notice that unhealthy behaviors actually strengthen trauma-based beliefs that aren't true. For example, self-neglect and risky and unhealthy behaviors tend to strengthen the belief that "It's OK for me to not take healthy care of myself," and self-harm tends to strengthen the belief that "It's OK for me to be hurt."

   Please note: Even if you do not believe it yet, it is not only OK but also *important to give yourself the care you need—and it is <u>not</u> OK for you to be hurt.* Believing that it is OK for you to be hurt is a trauma-based belief. When you find yourself thinking it is OK for you to be hurt, please be compassionate with yourself and work to manage and challenge these trauma-based thoughts.

3. Then consider several safe things that you are willing to commit to doing when that situation happens again. Your commitment can be anything you feel would be helpful and safe to you. Think about your growing list of healthy things you can do to help yourself when feeling too much or too little: Which of these might work best? Or you may think of other healthy ways to stay safe as you do this exercise. Add the ones you feel are most likely to be of help to the "Safe, healthy ways to help myself" sections.

4. Practice using these healthy ways to help yourself. After you've had some practice using healthy coping in these situations, complete the "short-term" and "longer-term" results sections for the "Results of responding in the new, healthy ways" sections. (See the tables above for examples.)

Healthy coping card

Situation	How I used to respond	Safe, healthy ways to help myself

Healthy coping results card

	Results of responding in the old, unsafe/unhealthy ways	Results of responding in the new, healthy ways
Short-term results		
Longer-term results		

Make a copy of your completed healthy coping card and healthy coping results card that you can carry with you. Consider making additional copies and hanging them on your refrigerator or on your bathroom mirror, saving them as photos on your phone, or placing them anywhere else you might often see them. You may also wish to keep creating healthy coping and healthy coping results cards as you become aware of situations that lead to difficulty for you; some people carry this "deck of cards" with them so the "deck is stacked" in their favor when they begin to have trouble because they can flip through the deck to find something that helps them. Finally, if you'd like, you can also recopy the cards from time to time to help yourself remember the new ways you're learning to help yourself.

Practice Exercise for Topic 15: The Cycle of Unhealthy Behavior and How to Break Out of It

We encourage you to continue to be on the lookout for your early warning signs so you can start practicing healthy coping using your warning signs safety plans or healthy coping cards as early as possible.

Noticing early warning signs and using healthy coping skills will help reduce how often "the last straw" events happen. If a "last straw" event happens anyway, a person who has been using skills will be better able to manage these situations well. Please also use healthy coping between the "last straw" and "unhealthy/unsafe behavior" steps, and remember that you can interrupt the cycle at any point.

If you do end up doing something unhealthy, please resist the temptation to tell yourself that you do not deserve better: That kind of discouraging self-talk keeps you trapped in the cycle. Instead, give yourself the care you need and start using healthy coping skills to interrupt the cycle. This will help keep you from developing increasing warning signs or getting stuck repeating old trauma-based thought patterns and behaviors.

Also, if you begin to do something unhealthy, remember that you can catch yourself and stop yourself from engaging in a lot of unhealthy behavior. Reducing the harm you do to yourself is better than doing more serious harm that is more likely to keep the cycle going.

Please also continue to practice getting your healthy needs met more safely and giving yourself compassionate care as you need it, especially when things are particularly challenging.

Don't forget to give yourself credit for all the work you are doing and each bit of progress! Each step you take makes a difference in helping your brain (and all of who you are) heal.

Step by step, you will get there!

References for Topic 15

Beck, J. (1995). *Cognitive therapy: Basics and beyond.* Guilford.

Boon, S., Steele, K., & van der Hart, O. (2011). *Coping with trauma-related dissociation: Skills training for patients.* W. W. Norton & Company.

Lewis, L., Kelly, K., & Allen, J. (2004). *Restoring hope and trust: An illustrated guide to mastering trauma.* Sidran Institute Press.

Najavits, L. M. (2002). *Seeking safety: A treatment manual for PTSD and substance abuse.* Guilford Press.

UNDERSTANDING AND REDUCING TRAUMA-RELATED REACTIONS

Information Sheet for Topic 16

In highly stressful/traumatic situations, people can find themselves "automatically" doing things without consciously choosing to do so. By practicing recovery-focused coping and getting healthy needs met safely, you can help yourself reduce these reactions and get better at noticing when you're at risk of having one—giving you the opportunity to choose how you would like to respond.

Reactions that people may have in response to highly stressful/overwhelming/traumatic situations

- **Flight/Avoidance:** The most common response is to attempt to escape/avoid such situations.
- **Fight/Interruption:** If it is not possible to avoid it, and it seems possible to stop it without making it worse, this becomes an option.
- **Freeze/Dissociation:** Dissociation (disconnecting from the here and now) is the escape when physical escape/avoidance or stopping the situation is not possible.
- **Submit/Submission:** To prevent worse things from happening, people may go along with what seems unavoidable/unstoppable. (This can include "please and appease" kinds of responses.)
- **Identify/Identification:** To increase a sense of control in situations where they do not seem to have any, people may see things from the perspective of the person with the power/control of the situation, dissociating their own thoughts and feelings.

How to reduce "automatically shifting" into these reactions when they are no longer necessary

- *Be compassionate with yourself and do not criticize or shame yourself for having these reactions.* These reactions are normal, understandable attempts to help you survive over-whelming situations that your brain chooses based on what it is aware of in the moment and what has helped in the past.

- It is especially important to be compassionate with yourself if these reactions are getting in the way of you getting and feeling safer: Changing how you do things takes lots of practice over time. Practice is hard to do without healthy self-compassion.
- Work to get your healthy needs met safely, and practice healing-focused coping. Notice what kinds of situations can lead to trauma-related reactions, and develop a plan to reduce the likelihood of shifting into such a reaction.
- Give yourself care and encouragement as you need it: Step by step, you'll get there!

EXERCISES FOR TOPIC 16: UNDERSTANDING AND REDUCING TRAUMA-RELATED REACTIONS

We hope you have been watching for your early warning signs and have been practicing healthy coping to interrupt cycles of unhealthy behavior. We also hope you have been continuing to practice getting your healthy needs met more safely and are being compassionate with yourself, especially when things are challenging.

In the information sheet for Topic 16, we talked about understanding and reducing trauma-related reactions, which can lead people to automatically do things without consciously choosing to do so. Please review this information before continuing on to the exercises below, which focus on helping you reduce trauma-related reactions.

Written Exercise for Topic 16: Understanding and Reducing Trauma-Related Reactions

In the information sheet for Topic 16, we emphasized that by practicing recovery-focused coping and getting your healthy needs met safely, you will eventually reduce how frequently you have these reactions when they are not necessary. Practicing recovery-focused coping and getting your healthy needs met safely will also make it easier to notice when you are starting to have a trauma-related reaction, giving you the opportunity to think about how you would like to respond.

This exercise will encourage you to identify the situations in which you are most likely to have a trauma-based reaction, as well as the signs that you might be having a trauma-related reaction that makes sense based on the past but doesn't fit the present situation. You can consider what healing-focused skills might be most helpful to help yourself manage these reactions.

As with all work in this program, make sure you are grounded before beginning. Please go at a pace that is manageable for you, taking breaks to ground and use healthy coping, paying attention to warning signs, and using your healthy coping cards and safety plans. Our goal is for you to get and feel safer. Please put safety and healthy coping first.

Are you grounded?

Let's start by identifying the situations in which you currently find yourself most likely to have one of these reactions.

Identifying trauma-related reaction triggers, warning signs, and healthy coping plans

1. In the "Trigger situation" column in the table below, list a situation where you are at risk of having a trauma-based reaction that does not fit the present.
   (If you find yourself wanting to write about more than one situation, select the one that feels most manageable to start with. Remember that you can always do more later, and/or that you

can talk to your therapist about these situations. You might work on this on different days this week so that you are pacing yourself.)

Trigger healthy coping plan

Trigger situation	Early warning signs	Healthy ways to help myself when I notice warning signs
		Orienting and anchoring to the present Separating past from present

2. Next, see if you can identify thoughts, emotions, physical sensations, and reactions you tend to have before a trauma-related reaction. List these signs that you might be starting to have a trauma-related reaction in the "Early warning signs" column.
3. Finally, consider what healthy coping skills in addition to grounding (orienting and anchoring to the present) and separating past from present might be helpful to slow or interrupt the trauma-related reaction. Write those in the "Healthy ways to help myself when I notice warning signs" column.

> *Note:* Trauma-related reactions often happen alongside crisis-level feelings; consider including aspects of your plan for managing crisis-level feelings (or the whole plan if it seems helpful) in your "healthy ways to help myself when I notice warning signs" plan.

"Inner war"

Sometimes people experience a sense of an inner war about what to do in response to reminders of trauma. This is linked with having multiple trauma-related reactions at the same time. If you experience inner war, please work to have compassion with yourself for each of these reactions: Each reaction makes sense as an attempt to reduce the impact of trauma or to avoid more harm.

For people who have parts

For people who have parts, it can be helpful to know that parts tend to take on one of the five trauma-related reactions described in the information sheet for Topic 16. It is also important to know that each part is reacting out of fear of further trauma and is acting in the way they believe is most likely to result in the least amount of trauma. (This is often not easily noticed by other parts, however.)

Practice Exercise for Topic 16: Understanding and Reducing Trauma-Related Reactions

We encourage you to keep watching for early warning signs to start practicing healthy coping and to follow the plan you have made for managing trauma-related reactions. With practice, noticing early warning signs and using healthy coping skills will reduce how often seemingly "last straw" events and trauma-related reactions happen; it will also make it easier to reduce their impact if they do happen.

Please continue to work toward getting your healthy needs met more safely and giving yourself compassionate care as you need it, especially when things are challenging.

Don't forget to give yourself credit for all the work you are doing and each bit of progress! Each effort makes a difference in helping your brain (and all of who you are) heal.

> *Remember:*
>
> As you continue through the program, strive to integrate what you've been learning into your daily routines. We recognize that this is much easier said than done, so please be patient with yourself as you work toward getting better and better at:
> - grounding;
> - separating past from present;
> - getting your healthy needs met safely;
> - planning for difficult situations;
> - recognizing early warning signs;
> - giving yourself the care you need to help you manage difficult situations, break the cycle of unhealthy behavior, reduce trauma-related reactions, and heal trauma's impact on the brain;
> - being curious about (and challenging) potential trauma-based thoughts; and
> - noticing and giving yourself credit for progress.

Congratulations on completing the fourth module! Step by step, you're getting there!

In the modules that follow, we'll offer additional information and skills to help you keep making progress toward getting and feeling safer.

Addressing Trauma-Based Thinking

This module focuses on learning how to identify and reduce trauma-based thinking.

This module will help you learn:

- about trauma-based thoughts as a common symptom of trauma
- how to identify trauma-based thoughts
- how to reduce trauma-based thoughts.

This module will help you practice:

- identifying trauma-based thoughts
- noticing evidence against trauma-based thoughts
- shifting from trauma-based thoughts to healing-focused thinking.

This difficult, important work builds on all you've already done as part of this program. Taking the time to do the work involved in reducing trauma-based thoughts can go a long way toward getting and feeling safer. Please give yourself the care you need as you do this work.

SHIFTING FROM TRAUMA-BASED THOUGHTS TO HEALING-FOCUSED THINKING

Information Sheet for Topic 17

People who have experienced trauma often have trauma-based thoughts about themselves, others, and the world. Having these kinds of thoughts after experiencing trauma is understandable—and can interfere with noticing when you are safer, giving yourself the care you need, and meeting your healthy needs in safe ways. To help yourself make progress toward getting and feeling safer, work to shift trauma-based thoughts to healing-focused thinking.

What should I know about trauma-based thoughts?

- Trauma-based thoughts are a common trauma-related symptom. *(If you have them, it is not your fault.)*
- Trauma-based thoughts are thoughts that are not true but that feel true based on traumatic experiences.
- Trauma-based thoughts typically happen when you are reminded of something emotionally overwhelming from your past.
- To help yourself heal, is important to actively work to notice any "evidence" that goes against trauma-based thoughts *without* minimizing 1) anything in the present that is not OK or 2) that these kinds of reactions make sense when something in the present has reminded you of something difficult from the past.
- Noticing evidence against trauma-based thoughts takes *lots* of active effort and practice. This is because how we think shapes what we notice when we look at the world (and ourselves):
  - We tend to notice and give more weight to evidence that fits or supports what we already think or believe.
  - We tend to *not* notice evidence that goes against our existing thoughts, or, if we do, we often discount or minimize its relevance or importance.

To help yourself shift from trauma-based thoughts to healing-focused thinking, notice your reactions with curiosity and self-compassion.

What are signs I might be having trauma-based thoughts?

Without minimizing anything in the present that is not OK, get curious when:

- you are having an intense or overwhelming emotion
- a situation feels like or "just like" something from the past
- you feel you must do something urgently
- you are having an intensely negative reaction to someone, or
- you are having intensely negative thoughts about yourself.

What are the steps to shift trauma-based thoughts to healing-focused thinking?

If you find yourself recognizing that you are having a trauma-based thought:

1. **Give yourself credit!** It is not easy to notice these kinds of thoughts, especially since they often accompany trauma-related reactions.

2. **Give yourself compassion and the care you need.** Remember that it is very understandable to have trauma-based thoughts when you have a history of trauma.

3. **Collect any evidence** that helps you notice and remember that this trauma-based thought is not true (or not always true).

4. **Make a list** of any trauma-based thought that you have been able to notice—if only once—is not true. Keep collecting evidence that helps you recognize the thought is not true.

5. **Create recovery-focused thoughts to replace trauma-based ones, and collect evidence that the healing-focused thoughts are true.**

Remember: Each time you work to address trauma-based thoughts helps your brain get better at noticing when you are safer; trim fear pathways; and build new, calm, healthy pathways.

    Each effort you make (whether you notice or not!) **helps toward your goal!**

EXERCISES FOR TOPIC 17: SHIFTING FROM TRAUMA-BASED THOUGHTS TO HEALING-FOCUSED THINKING

We hope you have been watching for your early warning signs and that you have been practicing healthy coping to interrupt cycles of unhealthy behavior and manage trauma-related reactions. We also hope you have been continuing to practice getting your healthy needs met safely and are being compassionate with yourself, especially when things are challenging.

In the information sheet for Topic 17, we talked about shifting from trauma-based thoughts to healing-focused thinking. Please review the information sheet before continuing on to the exercises below, which focus on helping you make this shift.

Written Exercises for Topic 17: Shifting from Trauma-Based Thoughts to Healing-Focused Thinking

Trauma-based thoughts are thoughts that are not true but that feel true based on traumatic experiences. In the information sheet, we emphasized that having trauma-based thoughts after experiencing trauma is understandable—and can interfere with giving yourself the care you need and meeting your healthy needs in safe ways. Working to shift trauma-based thoughts to healing-focused thinking is a crucial (and understandably difficult) part of helping yourself get and feel safer.

In the exercises for Topic 11, you practiced identifying trauma-based thoughts. You also practiced collecting evidence that these thoughts were unfair/untrue by listing things you noticed "at least once that suggest the thought is not true."

The exercise that follows will build on that work by reviewing some common thoughts that can feel true due to trauma (but aren't true or fair) and offering examples of healing-focused thoughts that are more accurate and fair.

As with all work in this program, make sure you are grounded before beginning. Please go at a pace that is manageable for you, taking breaks to ground and use healthy coping, paying attention to warning signs, and using your healthy coping and safety plans as necessary. Our goal is for you to get and feel safer—please put safety and healthy coping first.

Are you grounded? If yes, let's start.

Written exercise 1: Identifying healing-focused thoughts to challenge trauma-based thoughts

This exercise offers examples of how to challenge trauma-based thoughts with healing-focused thoughts.

1. Please read the examples of "Trauma-based thoughts" in the table below.[1] Mark any examples that you believe (or have believed) about yourself with an X.

---

[1] Exercises informed by Najavits, 2002, p. 216, and Boon et al., 2011, pp. 232–235.

(Note that if you have parts, different parts may have different thoughts. Please try to be curious about different parts' thoughts.)

2. Read the examples of "Healing-focused thoughts" in the right-hand column of the table. Notice that **healing-focused thoughts *do not ignore difficulties or negative information*.** Unlike trauma-based thoughts, however, **healing-focused thoughts *do include mention of positives and strengths*.** Healthy, **healing thoughts** are *self-compassionate, fair* thoughts.

3. Identify a healing-focused thought for each trauma-based thought you endorsed. *(The thought most helpful to you may not always be the one directly to the right of the trauma thought you marked with an X.)*

Trauma-based thoughts *(These thoughts <u>are not true</u> but <u>feel true</u> based on traumatic experiences.)*	Healing-focused thoughts *(These thoughts are more fair and healthy.)*
"I'm no good." "People can see how awful I am, so I have to stay away from them."	"I've been hurt. I have difficulties from being hurt, but trauma survivors are not bad. I'm not bad. I deserve help and healing, just like all trauma survivors deserve help and healing."
"Nobody would like me if they really got to know me." "Everybody else is better than me."	"I have strengths and weaknesses, like everyone." "I am working toward healing and making improvements in my life." "I don't have to be perfect to be OK, worthy of care, or deserving of safety."
"It is all my fault I was treated badly." "I deserved to be hurt. If I had been a better child, the abuse wouldn't have happened, or at least it would not have happened as often."	"No one deserves to be hurt, not even me." "I have made mistakes like all people do, but I didn't deserve to be hurt."
"Others will always hurt me." "Nobody can be trusted." "People will always hate me, hurt me, or abandon me."	"Although it's true that some people have hurt me in the past, not all people hurt other people. Not everyone will hurt me." "Not all people are unsafe. I will learn to pay attention to (and not ignore) signs that someone is unsafe. I will learn to protect myself in relationships. This may mean that I will have to change or end some relationships. I will work to keep healthy boundaries in relationships."
"What I need does not matter."	"I deserve to get my healthy needs met safely. It is OK and healthy to expect respect and to not stay in situations where I am not being respected."
"It's not OK to express what I need or to speak up to others if I don't like something."	"To build a healthy relationship, it is important to be able to express my needs and say when I do not like something. It is healthy and strong to be able to say 'no' to people if what they want is not good for me. If I begin to feel it is not OK to say 'no' in a relationship, that is a warning sign to pay close attention to the relationship. I need to think about whether the person is healthy for me. If I am concerned that I may be in an unsafe or unhealthy relationship, I will protect myself and talk to my therapist."

"Relationships always include exploitation and harm, so I will always get harmed if I get in a relationship. The only way to protect myself is to avoid relationships."	"Relationships that include exploitation and harm are *unsafe* relationships. *Healthy* relationships are based on mutual caring. In healthy relationships, both people's healthy needs get met safely. It is important to stay away from unhealthy relationships. All people need healthy relationships."
"I have to hurt myself before someone hurts or scares me. They will not hurt me if I am already hurt."	"Hurting myself only hurts me. It does not protect me from harm. If I am afraid that I am in a relationship with an unsafe person, I will protect myself and talk to my therapist about the situation."
"I have to give in to what I think others want so they do not hurt or leave me."	"Feeling that I need to do something because I am afraid someone will hurt me is a warning sign. I need to pay close attention to the relationship if I am feeling like this. Is there evidence that the person is unsafe? If I am concerned about being in an unsafe relationship, I will protect myself and talk to my therapist."
"I have to hurt or scare others before they can hurt or scare me."	"Hurting or scaring others would be doing to others what has been done to me. I don't want that. If I am concerned about being in an unsafe relationship, I will protect myself and talk to my therapist. If I worry that I may scare or harm someone else, I will talk to my therapist about it."

Written exercise 2: Identifying and addressing your trauma-based thoughts

This exercise encourages you to do the difficult work of noticing and addressing *your* trauma-based thoughts.

1. Review the "What Are Signs I Might Be Having Trauma-Based Thoughts?" section in the information sheet for Topic 17. Which thoughts come to mind as you review these signs? (Thoughts you've already listed as potential trauma-based thoughts in the exercises for Topic 11 on pp. 84–85? Other thoughts?) Please list these in the left-hand column of the table on page 145 as potential trauma-based thoughts.

2. To help yourself notice thinking mistakes that might be leading you to believe trauma-based thoughts, review Topic 4's table that lists "Thinking mistakes that we're all at risk of making" (see p. 36). Check each potential trauma-based thought that you write in the table below against that list: Is it possible that this thought is the result of one or more of these thinking mistakes? (For example, Is my thinking extreme? Am I ignoring important aspects? Am I overgeneralizing? Am I jumping to conclusions without looking at all the evidence? Am I mislabeling?)

3. If you find yourself having difficulty noticing or remembering evidence against trauma-based thoughts, review Topic 11's suggestions for collecting evidence against trauma-based thoughts. (Refer back to p. 86.)

4. Work to develop a healing-focused thought for each trauma-based thought you identify in the table below.

> *TIPS:*
>
> - This is difficult work that requires practice over time. Please be patient with yourself and give yourself the care you need as you do this work.
> - This is an exercise we recommend coming back to when you notice signs you might be having trauma-based thoughts.
> - If you have difficulty identifying trauma-based thoughts, deciding whether a thought is trauma-based, or developing healing-focused thoughts, consider talking to your therapist about the thought you are struggling with so you can work on this together.

Trauma-based thoughts *(These thoughts <u>are not true</u> but <u>feel true</u> based on traumatic experiences.)*	Healing-focused thoughts *(These thoughts are more fair and healthy.)*

Practice Exercise for Topic 17: Shifting from Trauma-Based Thoughts to Healing-Focused Thinking

Select three healing-focused thoughts you would like to begin to work on for the practice exercise, and list them on the table on page 145.

1. Look for "evidence" that the healing thought is accurate or true. It is OK if the healing thought does not always feel true. Look for evidence or signs that it is *sometimes* true. Remind yourself that if we are convinced something is true, we tend to only see evidence that supports the old (trauma-based) thought. Notice evidence that contradicts trauma-based thoughts. Notice evidence that supports healing thoughts.

2. Please also work on noticing when you are having untrue trauma-based thoughts—and give yourself credit anytime you "catch" these thoughts! It is difficult and important to notice when you are caught in trauma thinking.

3. As you come up with challenges to trauma-based thoughts that you intellectually know to be true, write them down whether or not you believe them emotionally. Consider reading over the "Evidence that supports the healing-focused thought" (things you've noticed at least once that suggest the thought is not true) multiple times a day, even when things are going well. (See p. 147.)

4. Allow yourself to be curious and to pay close attention to all of your experiences. Notice neutral and good experiences. Let yourself notice when you or other people are being trustworthy or kind. We are not encouraging you to ignore aspects of your experience. Instead, we are encouraging you to pay attention to experiences you may have not noticed before.

Over time, you will notice more evidence against unfair, untrue, and unhelpful thoughts and begin to notice different experiences of yourself. You will notice experiences that will help create more fair and helpful thoughts that will make it easier to get and feel safer.

Be compassionate with yourself as you do this very challenging work. This will take active effort and lots of practice. Please also continue to practice getting your healthy needs met more safely and giving yourself compassionate care as you need it (including using your coping and safety plans), especially when things are challenging. Give yourself lots of credit for doing this difficult work! You can feel proud about working hard to improve your safety and health.

Each step you are taking makes a difference in helping your brain (and all of who you are) heal. Step by step, you will get there!

Healing-focused thoughts *(These thoughts are fair and healthy.)*	Evidence that supports the healing-focused thought

References for Topic 17

Boon, S., Steele, K., & van der Hart, O. (2011). *Coping with trauma-related dissociation: Skills training for patients.* W. W. Norton & Company.

Najavits, L. M. (2002). *Seeking safety: A treatment manual for PTSD and substance abuse.* Guilford Press.

MAKING THE DECISION TO GET HEALTHIER AND SAFER

Information Sheet for Topic 18

Many people who have difficulty taking healthy care of themselves have a hard time making the decision to get healthier and safer in how they live.

Why can it be so hard to make a decision to get healthier and safer?

Making a decision to get healthier and safer can be difficult if:

- Risky, unhealthy, or unsafe behaviors are the way someone is used to getting a sense of relief.
- The person has not yet noticed how these behaviors keep them stuck in a cycle of feeling too much or too little, using unhealthy behavior to get relief, and then feeling unsafe and/ or too much or too little again.
- Trauma-based thoughts are making it hard to believe they deserve to be healthy and safe.
- They are still learning how to relate to themselves with healthy self-compassion.
- They do not have enough practice using healthy ways of helping themselves when feeling too much or too little.

How can I help myself make a decision to get healthier and safer?

- Keep applying and practicing the information shared in this program at a pace that works for you. Revisit information sheets and exercises.
- Consider deciding to be healthy and safe "one day at a time." Each day you get your healthy needs met safely helps your brain develop new, healthy pathways.
- Consider making a list of reasons to get healthier and safer (*i.e., how/why getting and feeling healthier and safer would help you*).
- Consider making a list of reasons *not* to do unhealthy behaviors (*i.e., the negative effects and consequences of doing risky, unhealthy, or unsafe behaviors*).
- Keep adding to these lists as you notice new reasons.
- Talk about this topic with your therapist.
- When you feel you are ready, make a commitment to work hard to get healthier and safer.
- If you make mistakes along the way, do not shame or harshly criticize yourself. Instead, give yourself the care you need to help yourself recommit to breaking the cycle of unhealthy behavior.

EXERCISES FOR TOPIC 18: MAKING THE DECISION TO GET HEALTHIER AND SAFER

We hope you have been noticing the evidence for healing-focused thoughts and challenges to trauma-based beliefs.

We also hope you have been continuing to practice getting your healthy needs met more safely and you are being compassionate with yourself, especially when things are challenging.

In the information sheet for Topic 18, we discussed some of the factors involved in feeling committed to getting healthier and safer and why this can sometimes be very difficult.

Please review the information sheet before continuing on to the exercises below, which focus on helping you examine factors involved in this decision.

Written Exercises for Topic 18: Making the Decision to Get Healthier and Safer

As with all work in this program, make sure you are grounded before beginning this work. Go at a pace that is manageable for you, taking breaks to ground and use healthy coping, paying attention to warning signs, and using your healthy coping and safety plans as necessary. Our goal is for you to get and feel safer—please put safety and healthy coping first.

Are you grounded? If yes, let's continue.

Written exercise 1: Factors involved in making the decision

There are a number of factors that can make it easier—or harder—to commit to getting healthier and safer, and understanding these factors can help you notice what kind of work will be most helpful.

With this in mind, if you find yourself having difficulty feeling committed to getting and feeling safer (including working to reduce risky, unhealthy, or unsafe behaviors), please review the list of "Reasons It Can Be Hard to Commit to Getting Healthier and Safer" below. For each statement, rate the degree it is true for you.

Reasons it can be hard to commit to getting healthier and safer

1. 1. Risky, unhealthy, or unsafe behaviors are the way I get a sense of relief.

    0%   10   20   30   40   50   60   70   80   90   100%

    (never true)   (always true)

2. I do not see evidence that risky, unhealthy, or unsafe behaviors keep me stuck in a cycle of feeling too much or too little.

    0%   10   20   30   40   50   60   70   80   90   100%

    (never true)   (always true)

3. I do not believe I deserve to be healthier and safer.

    0%   10   20   30   40   50   60   70   80   90   100%

    (never true)   (always true)

---

4. I do not relate to myself with self-compassion.

	0%	10	20	30	40	50	60	70	80	90	100%

(never true)   *(always true)*

5. I am not able to effectively use healing-focused coping skills yet.

	0%	10	20	30	40	50	60	70	80	90	100%

(never true)   *(always true)*

Review your answers; the more statements you tend to agree with, the more difficult it can be to commit to getting and feeling safer. Consider sharing your results with your therapist—and we hope the following suggestions can be of help:

- If you rated reason number 1 highly, it is important to find healthy ways to help yourself when you're feeling too much or too little; consider reviewing Module 1.
- If you rated reason number 2 highly, consider reviewing Topics 14 and 15.
- If your rating for number 3 is high, please know that you are suffering from unfair and untrue trauma-based beliefs (beliefs that are not true but feel true because of trauma). Please review the program's information sheets and exercises on trauma-based thoughts (Topics 11, 16, and 17) and talk to your therapist about this.
- It is very common for people who do not have enough practice being (or who have not been shown how to be) compassionate with themselves to have difficulty treating themselves with compassion. Consider reviewing Topics 10, 13, and 14. People who believe unfair trauma-based thoughts about themselves (like the statement in number 3) can also have difficulty relating to themselves with self-compassion. If this is true for you, continuing to work on trauma-based thoughts (Module 2 and Topics 11 and 17) will be helpful.
- Finally, if you rated number 5 highly, please remember that it takes lots of practice over time to learn how to do things differently. Keep practicing when you don't actively need the skills, and do your best to use the skills as soon as you can notice you might need them—you'll get there!

Written exercise 2: Ways my life could be better if I were feeling safer and getting my healthy needs met safely (including not doing risky/unhealthy/unsafe things)
For many people, it is easier to make progress toward getting and feeling safer when they keep the goals that are important to them in mind.

List *your reasons for wanting to get and feel safer* below, and add to this list as you become aware of more ways your life will be better as a result of getting and feeling safer.

(Some possibilities: If you use healthy ways to manage hard times and keep safer, you'll gradually be less distressed over time. Healthy coping will help you be able to participate in life in different and rewarding ways. If you have a hard time keeping yourself safe for yourself, you may also wish to remind yourself that using healthy coping and staying safe will help you be a better friend/parent/pet owner.)

_____

_____

_____

_____

_____

_____

_____

_____

_____

_____

_____

Written exercise 3: My reasons to <u>not</u> do risky/unhealthy/unsafe things
Many people find that staying mindful of their reasons *not* to do these behaviors helps them make progress.

List *your reasons for <u>not</u> doing these kinds of behaviors* below, and add to this list as you become aware of more reasons to not do these things.

(Review "How do these behaviors keep people stuck in a cycle of feeling unsafe?" in Topic 15's information sheet on pg. 122 and add any reasons from this section that you find meaningful. It may also be helpful to think of the consequences of doing risky/unhealthy/unsafe things. What negative

consequences have happened to you as a result of these behaviors? For example, how have they affected your relationships? Your health? Your finances? Your view of yourself? What other negative consequences has unhealthy behavior had on your life?)

_____

_____

_____

_____

_____

_____

_____

_____

_____

_____

_____

Written exercise 4: Committing to safety

Some people find they are better able to keep safe when they make a commitment to themselves to be safe. Some people find it helpful if they make a safety commitment with their therapist.

We encourage you to discuss with your therapist whether it would be helpful for you to make a safety agreement. For many people, making an agreement with themselves (including, if they have them, any/all parts or voices) helps them make a firmer commitment to being safe.

If you are ready to make such an agreement, the following example[2] may be useful to you and your therapist (but please work with your therapist to determine the right agreement for you):

_____

[2] Adapted from Sheppard Pratt Trauma Disorder Unit Patient handouts, v. 2013, informed by Braun, 1981; Kluft, 1983; Wilbur, 1982.

I promise that I will not hurt myself or anyone else, accidentally or on purpose. I promise that if I begin to have urges to break this safety agreement, I will use my warning signs safety plan (see Topic 14). If I can no longer keep safe, I will follow the steps my therapist and I have agreed upon, which may include calling a crisis hotline, calling my therapist, or going to the hospital.

If you are ready to make such an agreement, write your safety agreement below. If certain behaviors make you more likely to be unsafe, such as drinking too much or using drugs, it may help to include a commitment to limiting or not using drugs/alcohol.

_____

_____

_____

_____

_____

_____

_____

Practice Exercise for Topic 18: Making the Decision to Get Healthier and Safer

Keep applying and practicing the information shared in this program at a pace that works for you. If you've been having difficulty making the decision to get healthier and safer, revisit the information you found helpful related to "Reasons it can be hard to commit to getting healthier and safer" (e.g., trauma-based thoughts,[3] self-compassion,[4] the cycle of unhealthy behavior[5]), and consider talking about these topics with your therapist. When you feel you are ready, make a commitment to work hard to get healthier and safer.

To help remember how this difficult work will help, review and add to your list of "Ways my life could be better if I were feeling safer and getting my healthy needs met safely" (p. 151) and your list of reasons *not* to do unhealthy behaviors (p. 152) (i.e., the negative effects and consequences of doing risky, unhealthy, or unsafe behaviors).

---

[3] Topics 11, 16, and 17.
[4] Topic 10.
[5] Topic 15.

If making a commitment to being safe is very difficult for you, consider deciding to be healthy and safe "one day at a time." Each day you get your healthy needs met safely helps your brain develop new, healthy pathways.

If you make mistakes along the way, do not shame or harshly criticize yourself. Instead, give yourself the care you need to help yourself recommit to breaking the cycle of unhealthy behavior.

Remember to give yourself credit for all the work you are doing and each bit of progress! Each effort makes a difference in helping your brain (and all of who you are) heal.

Remember:

As you continue through the program, strive to integrate what you've been learning into your daily routines. We recognize that this is much easier said than done, so please be patient with yourself as you work toward getting better and better at:

- grounding
- separating past from present
- getting your healthy needs met safely
- planning for difficult situations
- recognizing early warning signs
- giving yourself the care you need to manage difficult situations, break the cycle of unhealthy behavior, reduce trauma-related reactions, and heal trauma's impact on the brain
- recognizing and addressing trauma-based thoughts
- noticing and giving yourself credit for progress.

Congratulations on completing the fifth module! Step by step, you're getting there!

In the modules that follow, we'll offer additional information and skills to help you keep making progress toward getting and feeling safer.

References for Topic 18

Braun, B. (1981). Hypnosis for multiple personalities. In H. Wain (Ed.), *Clinical hypnosis in medicine* (pp. 209–217). Year Book Publishers.

Kluft, R. P. (1983). Hypnotic crisis intervention in multiple personality, *American Journal of Clinical Hypnosis*, 26(2), 73–83.

Trauma Disorders Program, Sheppard Pratt Health System—Patient handouts, v. 2013.

Wilbur, C. (May, 1982). Psychodynamic approaches to multiple personality. Paper presented at the Annual Meeting of the American Psychiatric Association, Toronto, Canada.

Getting and Feeling Safer, Part 2

This module focuses on learning more ways to help yourself recognize, interrupt, and reduce things that get in the way of and getting and feeling safer.

This module will help you learn:

- how to calm your alarm system
- about the window of tolerance
- how to help yourself get and feel safer by staying within and slowly expanding your window of tolerance.

This module will help you practice:

- collecting safer experiences
- doing things that help you calm your alarm system
- reducing exposure to unhealthy and retraumatizing experiences
- helping yourself when your risk of doing unhealthy or unsafe things is increasing.

This work builds on all you've already done as part of this program, and it will help you notice when you are safer and when you are at increased risk of doing something unhealthy or unsafe. Please give yourself the care you need as you do this work.

WORKING TO CALM YOUR ALARM SYSTEM

Information Sheet for Topic 19

It is important to help yourself heal the alarm system in your brain so you will not have to feel on "high alert" or surrounded by danger at all times.

How do I work to calm my alarm system?

- **Practice your orienting, anchoring, and other grounding skills to become more present in your current reality.** Take time to pay focused attention to the here and now. Orient yourself to the present by reminding yourself where you are, how old you are, and who is and who is not around you now. Anchor yourself in the present by using your five senses; by using any of the "101 Ways to Get Grounded"; and/or by describing in detail at least three things you can see, touch, hear, or smell in the here and now. Notice times where the situation around you is calm and/or not threatening—each time you do, you are helping your brain heal!

- **Take time throughout your day to notice how you are doing.** Check in with yourself several times a day, every day, to see how you are feeling. (If you have parts, this requires checking in with all parts of yourself.) Notice when you are doing OK, or even just a little bit better—it is important to recognize these experiences; each time you do, you are helping your brain heal!

- **If you recognize that you, or some part of you, is beginning to feel upset or distressed, it is important to take some time to give yourself the care you need and deal with those feelings in healthy ways.** If you are feeling upset, please try to remember to do deep breathing, to orient and anchor yourself to the present, and to use healing-focused coping skills to separate past from present and manage trauma-based thoughts.

- **If there is something unsafe or unhealthy in your life, it is crucial that you work to get safer in that part of your life.** Trauma-based thinking can sometimes get in the way, so keep using the skills you have been learning to help yourself shift toward a healing- and recovery-focused mindset.

- **If you have parts, help each other.** Those of you with parts may realize that some parts feel frightened all, or almost all, of the time. The more you can comfort and help your parts become oriented to and anchored in the here and now, the better you will feel. All parts of you benefit from helping the most vulnerable, hurt, and scared parts: Because all parts of a person share the same body and brain, when one part is having a hard time, it affects the whole person. As you help each part of yourself, it helps all parts (including the brain that all parts share) feel calmer and safer.

EXERCISES FOR TOPIC 19: WORKING TO CALM YOUR ALARM SYSTEM

We hope that you have been noticing the evidence for healing-focused thoughts and that you are keeping your commitment to get and feel safer (or working toward making that commitment). We also hope you have been continuing to practice getting your healthy needs met safely and are being compassionate with yourself, especially when things are challenging.

In the information sheet for Topic 19, we talked about how to help yourself calm your alarm system. Please review this information before continuing on to the exercises below, which focus on helping you put these recommendations into practice.

As with all work in this program, make sure you are grounded before beginning this work. Go at a pace that is manageable for you, taking breaks to ground and use healthy coping, paying attention to warning signs, and using your healthy coping and safety plans as necessary. Our goal is for you to get and feel safer—please put safety and healthy coping first.

Are you grounded? Let's start.

Written Exercises for Topic 19: Working to Calm Your Alarm System
Written exercise 1: Collecting safer experiences

As noted in the information sheet for Topic 19, an important part of helping yourself heal your brain's alarm system is noticing when things are safer, calm, not threatening, or OK.

One way to help yourself do this: Become an active "collector" of these kinds of experiences. Watch for experiences that are safer, calmer, not threatening, or OK, and make a list of them that you can review as "evidence" that safer situations really do exist.

TIP: As you go through your day, watch for, notice, and remember experiences that are safer, including neutral (i.e., neither good nor bad), calm, not threatening, boring, and OK experiences, and add these to the "Safer experiences" list below. Consider creating this kind of list each day. You can then review it at the end of the day and end of the week to help calm your alarm system by raising awareness of these experiences.

Safer experiences

_____

_____

_____

_____

_____

_____

_____

_____

_____

_____

_____

_____

_____

_____

_____

_____

TIP: To help yourself be best able to notice and collect safer experiences, focus on grounding and separating past from present.

A key component of being able to notice safer experiences is being grounded. It is very difficult to notice that the present is safer if you are not connected to the here and now. Working to get and stay grounded is the foundation for getting and feeling safer and calming your alarm system.

With this in mind, if you find yourself having difficulty staying connected to the here and now:

- Check in with yourself regularly to see if you need to orient to and anchor in the present.
- To help yourself track your progress, consider using the grounding check-sheet presented at the end of the exercises for Topic 2: Signs That You Are Starting to Get Ungrounded and Healthy Ways to Get Grounded (see p. 19).
- Review the grounding information sheets and exercises (in Module 1) again.

Significant difficulties with grounding can indicate difficulties with separating past from present. If you find yourself often feeling that the present is like or just like the past, please:

- Work to notice differences *without minimizing anything that is not OK* (i.e., do not minimize anything in the present that is unsafe or unhealthy), and
- Consider reviewing the separating past from present materials (in Module 2) again.

Written exercise 2: Reducing behaviors that get in the way of getting and feeling safer
It is hard to calm your alarm system if you are doing things that get in the way of your getting and feeling safer.

Review the table below to see a list of "Behaviors that get in the way of getting and feeling safer" and "Things that help me calm my alarm system."[1]

If you recognize that you do one or more of the "Behaviors that get in the way of getting and feeling safer," circle the corresponding recommendations in the "Things that help me calm my alarm system," and work to do those things instead.

Behaviors that get in the way of getting and feeling safer	Things that help me calm my alarm system
Not using healthy coping skills to get through difficult times	Using healthy coping skills
Not practicing grounding enough	Practicing grounding more often
Sleeping too much or too little	Getting a healthy amount of sleep (or staying in bed for only a healthy number of hours if I have trouble sleeping)
Isolating, withdrawing from people	Spending time with safe, supportive people
Skipping therapy, medical appointments	Going to therapy, making and keeping medical appointments as needed

---

[1] This exercise is adapted from an exercise by Lisa M. Najavits (2002, p. 194).

Behaviors that get in the way of getting and feeling safer	Things that help me calm my alarm system
Skipping work, school, or volunteering	Going to work, school, or volunteer job; communicating if need to miss for health reasons
Too much self-distraction using technology (e.g., surfing the web, social media, TV, video games)	Visiting with safe, supportive people or talking on the phone with them
Giving up on a healthy coping skill if it doesn't work right away	Keep practicing, trying, and using healthy coping skills even if I don't always get the quick relief I want. Repeatedly using healthy coping on tough days if the relief does not last.
Keeping overly busy so there is no time to take care of myself	Making my health a priority; taking time to take care of myself
Skipping meals or eating mostly junk food or fast food	Eating regular, healthy meals
Drinking too much alcohol	Drinking something soothing that is nonalcoholic like tea, coffee, or sparkling water
Not using medications as prescribed	Taking medication as prescribed without skipping doses or using too much
Staying up all night and sleeping all day, or having other irregular sleep habits	Keeping a regular, healthy bedtime and getting up at a regular time most days
Spending a lot of time trancing, spacing out, or otherwise dissociating	Working to use grounding techniques so I am rarely losing time due to dissociating
Repeating harsh, negative thoughts to myself; judging myself	When I criticize myself, recognizing it and trying to be more encouraging and compassionate with myself
Thinking about my problems or trauma over and over and over again so that I'm stuck in the thoughts	Gently interrupting myself and shifting my attention to something else when I notice I'm getting stuck in thinking too much about my problems or trauma
Telling myself that being healthy is too much work or that I don't deserve to get better	Keep trying. Keep reminding myself that I matter and deserve to get better, even when I don't feel like I matter or deserve it.
Getting into fights with people	Working to talk things out and get along with people. Or, if the relationship is unhealthy, working on protecting myself from harm.
Spending time with people who are discouraging of recovery, or who encourage me to use unhealthy coping	Spending time with people who encourage my recovery and use of healthy coping. Keeping good boundaries with people who are discouraging of my recovery.

Behaviors that get in the way of getting and feeling safer	Things that help me calm my alarm system
Keeping myself on high alert all the time on purpose because it seems like it will keep me safer	Recognizing that this is trauma-based thinking. Being on high alarm is a symptom of being traumatized and is unhealthy for my brain, body, and well-being when I am in safer situations. Reminding myself that I see situations and options more clearly when I'm grounded, and that this keeps me safer. Working on getting grounded and allowing myself to notice when situations are safer so that I can help my brain, body, and all of who I am heal.

Written exercise 3: Reduce exposure to unhealthy and retraumatizing experiences

It is also difficult to calm your alarm system if you are in unhealthy or unsafe relationships. Allow yourself to notice if you are involved in relationships that are unhealthy, somewhat unsafe, or even very unsafe.

People who have experienced trauma in their relationships sometimes have difficulty identifying signs of unsafe relationships. Review the list of signs of unhealthy and unsafe relationships below, noting any signs that apply to your relationships.

Signs of unhealthy and unsafe relationships include when someone is doing any of the following:[2]

- repeatedly being harshly critical of you or verbally aggressive with you
- regularly ignoring or invalidating your needs or concerns
- repeatedly blaming and/or shaming you about things they or others would not be blamed or shamed for
- encouraging risky, unhealthy, or unsafe behaviors
- discouraging healthy behaviors
- discouraging your spending time with safe friends/family members who are important to you
- physically hurting (or threatening to hurt) you or someone you love
- repeatedly lying to you
- using you (e.g., contacting you only when they need something, never paying their own way)
- making you do things you don't feel OK about.

If you have relationships that are unhealthy or unsafe for you, we strongly encourage you to talk to your therapist about this.

---

[2] Informed by a list by Lisa M. Najavits (2002, p. 278).

TIP: What do healthy relationships look like?

It may be helpful to know that healthy relationships are generally consistent with the principles of trauma-informed care.[3] Put another way, in healthy relationships, people are:

- *Physically and emotionally safe* (not being hurt or hurting someone else physically or emotionally)
- *Empowering* (encouraging each other to talk about their perspectives and preferences)
- *Collaborative* (working with each other to find solutions that work for all involved)
- *Supportive* (support one another as they work through difficulties and toward self-improvement)
- *Trustworthy* (they are honest and keep their word), and
- Striving to be *Mindful* of the impact of the past and gender and cultural biases.

Practice Exercise for Topic 19: Working to Calm Your Alarm System

We encourage you to follow the recommendations in the information sheet and written exercises for Topic 19 to calm your alarm system by:

- Working to stay grounded
- Collecting safer experiences
- Doing the things that help you calm your alarm system (instead of behaviors that get in the way of getting and feeling safer), and
- Reducing exposure to unhealthy and retraumatizing experiences.

Please also continue to practice getting your healthy needs met more safely and giving yourself compassionate care as you need it, especially when things are particularly challenging.

And don't forget to give yourself credit for all the work you are doing and each bit of progress! Each step you are taking makes a difference in helping your brain (and all of who you are) heal.

Step by step, you will get there!

References for Topic 19

Huang, L. N., Flatow, R., Biggs, T., Afayee, S., Smith, K., Clark, T., & Blake, M. (2014). *SAMHSA's concept of trauma and guidance for a trauma-informed approach*. Substance Abuse and Mental Health Services Administration.
Najavits, L. M. (2002). *Seeking safety: A treatment manual for PTSD and substance abuse*. Guilford Press.

---

[3] E.g., Huang et al., 2014.

FEELING TOO MUCH OR TOO LITTLE AND YOUR WINDOW OF TOLERANCE

Information Sheet for Topic 20

For people who have experienced trauma, the range of emotion and body sensation that is comfortable (i.e., the "window of tolerance") is typically very narrow, especially since trauma reminders can quickly lead people to feel too much or too little. In other words, trauma leads us to have overactive alarm systems that we need to work to calm and heal through the use of recovery-focused coping skills. Feeling too much or too little gets in the way of healing. Helping yourself stay within and heal your window of tolerance can make a big difference in helping yourself get and feel safer.

What is the window of tolerance?

The window of tolerance[4] (see Figure 6.1) is the range of emotional or physical sensation that feels manageable (i.e., not too much or too little).

People who have experienced trauma often have a narrow range of emotions and physical sensations that feel tolerable or manageable. This increases the risk for doing unsafe, risky, and/or unhealthy things and/or dissociation.

Why is it important to be aware of my window of tolerance?

Being aware of your window of tolerance helps you:
- Plan how to help yourself when you get outside your window of tolerance.
- Develop ways to notice risk of getting outside your window of tolerance.
- Identify things you can do to reduce the likelihood of getting outside your window of tolerance.

---

[4] Siegel, 1999; Ogden et al., 2006.

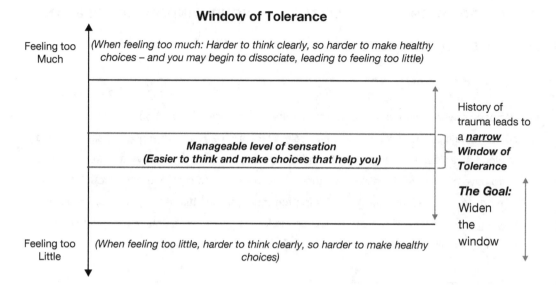

FIGURE 6.1. **The Window of Tolerance**

How can I notice risk of getting outside my window of tolerance?

- Start by describing what you notice about yourself when you are outside your window of tolerance. Then look for and describe the earliest signs of getting outside your window, and the changes you notice along the way.
- Keep those signs in mind as warning signs for getting outside your window.
- Consider developing gauge imagery (e.g., thermometers, pressure gauges, speedometers, or a series of colors) to help yourself track and notice where you are within your window.

How can I reduce the likelihood of getting outside my window of tolerance?

Identify healthy things you can do to help you stay in your window of tolerance when you are at risk of getting outside it.

How do I help myself heal my window of tolerance?

To heal and widen your window of tolerance, work toward:

- Staying within your window of tolerance by using recovery-focused coping skills (e.g., grounding, separating past from present, and containment) to help yourself heal your alarm system . . . and, when you are ready,

- Getting more comfortable with emotions and body sensations so they do not set off your alarm system when you are actually safer.

Be gentle, fair, and encouraging with yourself as you do this. Give yourself the care you need. Step by step, you'll get there!

EXERCISES FOR TOPIC 20: FEELING TOO MUCH OR TOO LITTLE AND YOUR WINDOW OF TOLERANCE

We hope you have been working to stay grounded, collecting safer experiences, doing the things that help you calm your alarm system, and reducing your exposure to unhealthy and retraumatizing experiences. We also hope you have been continuing to work toward getting your healthy needs met safely and that you are being compassionate with yourself and giving yourself the care you need, especially when things are challenging.

In the information sheet for Topic 20, we talked about the window of tolerance.[5] Please review the information sheet before continuing on to the exercises below, which focus on helping you identify your window of tolerance.

As with all work in this program, make sure you are grounded before beginning this work. Go at a pace that is manageable for you, taking breaks to ground and use healthy coping as you need to, paying attention to warning signs and using your healthy coping and safety plans. Our goal is for you to get and feel safer—please put safety and healthy coping first.

Are you grounded? Let's start.

Written Exercises for Topic 20: Feeling Too Much or Too Little and Your Window of Tolerance

For people who have experienced trauma, the range of emotion and body sensation that is comfortable (i.e., the window of tolerance) is typically very narrow, especially since trauma reminders can quickly lead people to feel too much or too little. In other words, trauma leads us to have overactive alarm systems that we need to work to calm and heal through the use of recovery-focused coping skills. Feeling too much or too little gets in the way of healing.

At the same time, our feelings and body sensations are signals to get us to pay attention to things that can help us get and stay safer. Emotions and body sensations are there to let us know when something is happening that needs our attention, so learning how to have a better relationship with emotions and body sensations—at a pace and in ways that feels manageable—is a very important aspect of healing. This kind of work often requires particular care, grounding, and thoughtful approaches to pacing so as not to move too fast. Please remember to give yourself the care you need as you do this work.

To help yourself get and feel safer, then, it is important to work toward:

- Staying within your window of tolerance by using recovery-focused coping skills (e.g., grounding, separating past from present, and containment) to help yourself heal your alarm system, and

---

[5] Siegel, 1999; Ogden et al., 2006.

- Helping yourself get more comfortable with emotions and body sensations so they do not set off your alarm system when you are actually safer.

It is important to work to stay within your window of tolerance using healthy coping skills. This will help you heal your alarm system. (Getting good at using healthy coping skills will also make it easier to expand/widen your window of tolerance later.)

Written exercise 1: Identifying the edges of your window of tolerance

It is easier to stay inside your window of tolerance if you are aware of the signs that you are starting to get outside of your window of tolerance. This exercise will guide you through the process of noticing these signs.[6]

Imagine that the numbers on the left side of Figure 6.2 represent a range of feeling, from 10 (*feeling very intense feelings or sensations*) to 0 (*uncomfortably numb*).

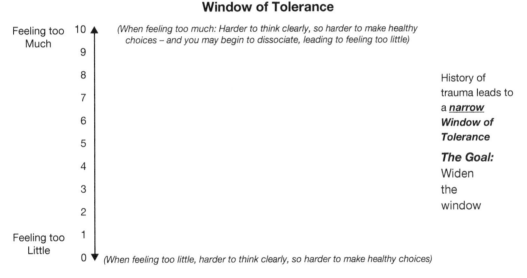

FIGURE 6.2. **Your Window of Tolerance**

1. What are the lowest and highest levels of feeling you feel comfortable having?

   (*These numbers represent the low and high ends of your window of tolerance.*)

   _____

2. How do you feel emotionally and what does your body feel like when you are experiencing feelings within your window of tolerance?

   _____

---

[6] Exercise adapted with permission from W.W. Norton & Company. Homework Sheet 18.1 & 18.2, pgs. 224-225, Boon, S., Steele, K., & van der Hart, O. (2011). Coping with trauma-related dissociation: Skills training for patients. New York, NY: W.W. Norton & Company.

(Possible examples: You may feel more OK, relaxed, energized, competent, in control, stable, settled.)

_____

_____

_____

_____

_____

3. How do you feel emotionally and what does your body feel like when you are feeling too much?

_____

_____

_____

_____

_____

_____

4. How do you feel emotionally and what does your body feel like when you are feeling too little?

_____

_____

_____

_____

_____

_____

_____

5. It is best to start using healthy coping skills as soon as you begin to feel outside your window of tolerance. At what levels of feeling *(low and high)* should you begin using skills to help manage your level of feelings?

_____

6. What does your body feel like at each of those levels? Describe the early signs of beginning to get beyond your window of tolerance.

(Remembering this will help you remember to begin to use skills at each of these levels.)

_____

_____

_____

_____

_____

_____

7. **If you have parts**, how do your parts' windows of tolerance compare to yours? Can some parts tolerate feeling more feelings? Do some parts have very little tolerance for feelings? Consider how you might work together to help all of who you are stay within a window of tolerance.

(You may find it helpful to talk to your therapist about this.)

_____

_____

_____

_____

_____

_____

_____

_____

_____

_____

_____

_____

_____

_____

_____

Written exercise 2: Healthy things to do when starting to feel too much or too little
Use the spaces below to list healthy things you can do to help yourself stay in (or get back in) your window of tolerance if you start to find yourself feeling too much or too little. (*For suggestions, see Topic 2: Signs That You Are Starting to Get Ungrounded and Healthy Ways to Get Grounded.*)

Healthy things to do when feeling too much:

_____

_____

_____

_____

_____

_____

Healthy things to do when feeling too little:

_____

_____

_____

_____

_____

_____

Practice Exercise for Topic 20: Feeling Too Much or Too Little and Your Window of Tolerance

We encourage you to work to be aware of when you start to get toward the edges of your window of tolerance and practice using the healthy things you have planned to use when starting to feel too much or too little.

Be sure to give yourself lots of credit each time you notice starting to feel too much or too little and each time you practice using healing-focused coping to help yourself get back into the window of tolerance!

Keep practicing getting your healthy needs met safely, giving yourself the care you need, and using healthy coping to break the cycle of unhealthy behavior. Be patient and compassionate with yourself. Lasting change takes practice and time. It is OK to go at a pace that is right for you. Keep at it!

Don't forget to give yourself credit for all the work you are doing and each bit of progress! Each step you take makes a difference in helping your brain (and all of who you are) heal.

Step by step, you will get there!

References for Topic 20

Boon, S., Steele, K., & van der Hart, O. (2011). *Coping with trauma-related dissociation: Skills training for patients.* W. W. Norton & Company.

Ogden, P., Minton, K., & Pain, C. (2006). *Trauma and the body: A sensorimotor approach to psychotherapy.* W. W. Norton & Company.

Siegel, D. J. (1999). *The developing mind: How relationships and the brain interact to shape who we are.* Guilford Press.

HELPING YOURSELF RECOGNIZE SIGNS THAT YOUR RISK OF DOING UNHEALTHY OR UNSAFE THINGS IS INCREASING

Information Sheet for Topic 21

> The window of tolerance is the range of emotional or physical sensation that feels manageable (not too much or too little). Helping yourself stay within and heal your window of tolerance can make a big difference in getting and feeling safer.

> *How can I notice increasing risk of doing something unhealthy or unsafe?*
>
> - Start by describing what you notice about yourself when you are outside your window of tolerance.
> - Then look for and describe the earliest signs of getting outside that window and the changes you notice along the way.
> - Keep those signs in mind as warning signs for getting outside that window.
> - Consider developing gauge imagery (e.g., thermometers, pressure gauges, speedometers, or a series of colors) to help yourself track and notice your current level of risk.

> *How can I reduce the risk of doing something unhealthy or unsafe?*
>
> - Think of the healthy things you can do to reduce your distress at each level of increasing warning signs.
> - Develop and follow a plan for how you will manage crisis-level feelings safely. This can and should include reaching out to treatment providers and/or emergency services for help as necessary/indicated.
> - Manage trauma-related thoughts, and work to shift trauma-related beliefs to healing-focused thinking.
> - Work toward getting your healthy needs met safely (including working to get and stay grounded when feeling too much or too little).
> - Work toward giving yourself the care you need as you need it.
> - Be gentle, fair, and encouraging with yourself as you do this. Step by step, you'll get there!

EXERCISES FOR TOPIC 21: HELPING YOURSELF RECOGNIZE SIGNS THAT YOUR RISK OF DOING UNHEALTHY OR UNSAFE THINGS IS INCREASING

We hope you have been working to be aware of when you start to get toward the edges of your window of tolerance and practicing using the healthy things you have planned to use when feeling too much or too little. Be sure to give yourself lots of credit each time you notice starting to feel too much or too little and each time you practice using healing-focused coping to help yourself get back into the window of tolerance.

We also hope you are working to stay grounded, collecting safer experiences, doing the things that help you calm your alarm system (instead of things that get in the way of getting and feeling safer), and reducing your exposure to unhealthy and retraumatizing experiences.

In the information sheet for Topic 21, we talked about helping yourself when your risk of doing unhealthy or unsafe things is increasing. Please review the information sheet before continuing on to the exercises below, which focus on how to notice and help yourself when you are at increasing risk of doing something unhealthy or unsafe.

As with all work on this program, make sure you are grounded before beginning this work. Go at a pace that is manageable for you, taking breaks to ground, and use healthy coping as you need to.

Are you grounded? Let's start.

Written Exercise for Topic 21: Helping Yourself Recognize Signs That Your Risk of Doing Unhealthy or Unsafe Things Is Increasing

Developing a plan to keep yourself in your window of tolerance
Trauma leads us to have overactive alarm systems that we need to work to calm and heal through the use of recovery-focused coping skills. Helping yourself stay within and heal your window of tolerance can make a big difference in getting and feeling safer. Feeling too much or too little gets in the way of healing.

In the last exercise, we encouraged you to work to identify the edges of your window of tolerance. In this exercise, we encourage you to work toward identifying the earliest signs of getting outside that window and the changes you notice along the way.

Below you will find a table that asks you to describe the:

- Thoughts,
- Feelings, and
- Body sensations

that you experience at five levels of distress, ranging from low or no distress to being in crisis.[7] When completing these descriptions, think about times when:

1. You are feeling as calm and OK as you have ever felt (*if it helps, think about neutral/OK experiences you have been collecting*).
2. You are just beginning to get anxious or stressed.
3. Your stress/anxiety is increasing.
4. You are starting to approach the edge of your window of tolerance.
5. You are at (or over) the edge of your window of tolerance, and it feels like you are in crisis and at high risk of doing risky/unhealthy/unsafe behaviors.

The table also has a column for you to list healthy things you can do to help yourself lower your distress or interrupt an increase in distress at each level ("Healthy coping/Safety plan"). When completing this column, to save space and make the table easy to read, some people find it helpful to assume that they are adding healthy things at each level. (For example: They may list grounding, separating past from present, and containment as healthy things they can do at Level 1 to help them stay feeling calm and OK, and then know that they will be using these skills at each higher level, too.)

Please talk to your therapist about this plan, including about when it is time to reach out to them and/or call emergency services.

The goal of this exercise is to develop a plan that helps you get and feel safer when you notice increasing levels of distress. As you do this work, please put safety and healthy coping first. Pay attention to warning signs, and use your healthy coping and safety plans as necessary.

Are you grounded? Continue on.

---

[7] Adapted from Sheppard Pratt Patient handouts, v. 2013.

Plan to keep myself in my window of tolerance

Level	Thoughts	Feelings	Body sensations	Healthy coping/ Safety plan
1 *(Feeling as calm and OK as you have ever felt)*				
2 *(Just beginning to get anxious or stressed)*				
3 *(Stress/anxiety is increasing)*				
4 *(Starting to approach edge of window of tolerance)*				
5 *(At/over edge of window of tolerance, feels like you are in crisis and at high risk of doing something risky/unhealthy/ unsafe)*				

Practice Exercise for Topic 21: Helping Yourself Recognize Signs That Your Risk of Doing Unhealthy or Unsafe Things Is Increasing

Practice using your plan to keep yourself in your window of tolerance. Be aware of when you start to get toward the edges of each level of distress, and practice using the healthy things you have planned to use at that level.

Be sure to give yourself lots of credit each time you notice the level of distress you are feeling and each time you practice healthy coping to help yourself stay or get back into your window of tolerance.

Be patient and compassionate with yourself. Lasting change takes practice and time. It is OK to go at a pace that is right for you. Keep at it!

And don't forget to give yourself credit for all the work you are doing and each bit of progress along the way. Each step you are taking makes a difference in helping your brain (and all of who you are) heal.

Remember:

As you continue through the program, strive to integrate what you've been learning into your daily routines. We recognize that this is much easier said than done, so please be patient with yourself as you work toward getting better and better at:

- getting your healthy needs met safely
- noticing where you are in your window of tolerance
- grounding
- separating past from present
- planning for difficult situations
- recognizing early warning signs
- giving yourself the care you need to help yourself manage difficult situations, break the cycle of unhealthy behavior, reduce trauma-related reactions, and heal trauma's impact on the brain
- recognizing and addressing trauma-based thoughts
- noticing and giving yourself credit for progress.

Congratulations on completing the sixth module! Step by step, you're getting there!

In the modules that follow, we'll offer additional information and exercises that build on all the work you've been doing to keep making progress toward getting and feeling safer.

Reference for Topic 21

Trauma Disorders Program, Sheppard Pratt Health System—Patient handouts, v. 2013.

MODULE 7

Improving Your Relationship with Emotions, Body Sensations, and Aspects of Self

Trauma can dramatically change the range of emotions and physical sensations that feel comfortable, OK, or manageable. People who have experienced trauma often feel too much or too little emotion/body sensations for reasons that are not always clear to them, and traumatic experiences can lead people to believe that certain feelings are not OK—or that having emotions is not OK. These situations can lead people to not want—or even to be afraid of—their emotions and body sensations. In addition, they may never have learned how to have a healthy relationship with their emotions, body sensations, or themselves.

At the same time, it is difficult to get and feel safer without a healthy relationship with your emotions, body, and all of who you are. This module will help you work toward manageably developing healthy relationships with these aspects of your experience and yourself to help all of who you are get and feel safer.

This module will help you learn:

- how to help your feelings help you
- why naming feelings can be so difficult
- <u>your</u> reasons for developing healthier relationships with your feelings
- ways to identify what you are feeling
- what your feelings are trying to help you notice
- how to work toward better relationships with your feelings and all of who you are.

This module will help you practice:

- noticing what you feel comfortable feeling, and which feelings might be helpful and manageable to work on having better relationships with
- noticing how you are currently relating to your feelings
- safely noticing and naming feelings
- building better relationships with your feelings and all aspects of who you are.

This difficult, important work builds on all you've already done as part of this program, and it represents another meaningful set of steps toward getting and feeling safer. Please give yourself the care you need as you do this work.

HOW TO HELP YOUR FEELINGS HELP YOU

Information Sheet for Topic 22

Developing healthy relationships with your emotions (feelings) and body sensations is an important part of getting and feeling safer. Emotions and body sensations help us notice when it feels like something important is happening, and they encourage us to do something that will help us.

BUT: We may not be noticing what is actually happening, especially if we are not connected to the here and now.

Why might feelings feel scary, bad, or wrong?

- People who have experienced trauma can feel too much or too little emotion and/or body sensations for reasons that are not always clear to them. This can include "flashbacks" of emotions or sensations related to trauma.
- Traumatic experiences can lead people to believe that certain feelings are not OK—or that having emotions is not OK.
- Trauma can dramatically change the range of emotions and physical sensations that feel comfortable, OK, or manageable.

These situations can lead people to not want or even to be afraid of their emotions and body sensations.

Why might people want to work toward being more comfortable with having and recognizing their feelings and body sensations?

- **To be safer/reduce the risk of getting hurt.** Because feelings give us important information about the world around us, being in touch with your feelings helps you get and stay safer. For example, our feelings can help us notice if someone is reliable and caring, or if they are unpredictable, or frightening, or insensitive.
- **To keep us healthy.** Being aware of when our body is trying to tell us we need to do something different than what we're currently doing can help us get and stay healthy. If we can tune in to our bodies, including the sensations they send, our bodies can tell us if we are thirsty and need to drink something, hungry and need to eat something, full and need to stop eating or drinking, tired and need to sleep, tense or restless and need some exercise, or sick or injured and need to see a doctor.

- **To be less overwhelmed.** Learning to pay attention to feelings in healthy, manageable ways will make you less susceptible to getting overwhelmed, dissociated, or tempted to use unhealthy ways to manage feelings.
- **To have more enjoyable lives.** People who have learned how to be comfortable with their feelings are better able to deeply enjoy their lives, including watching movies, listening to music, enjoying food, having meaningful relationships, and so on. Part of what makes these experiences enjoyable is the feelings they bring. People who have learned how to be comfortable with their bodies are able to enjoy when their bodies feel strong, capable, and healthy.

If we can learn how to listen to our emotions and our bodies, there is much wisdom we can learn. (This may be the opposite of how you currently experience your body and feelings.)

How can I develop a healthy relationship with my emotions?

Work toward relating to yourself with **curiosity** and **compassion**.

Relate to your emotions with **curiosity**. Ask yourself:

- What am I feeling, and why might I be feeling this way?
- Is there something I am missing? (Am I grounded/connected to the here and now?)
- Are there things I am not paying attention to? Am I being fair?
- What can I do that will best help me toward having the life I want?

Relate to yourself with **compassion**. Remind yourself:

- Feelings always make sense based on what we *think* is happening/has happened/might happen.
- It is difficult to notice (and easy to minimize) things that do not fit what you are thinking and feeling. Give yourself lots of credit if you can notice something you had not noticed before!
- Give yourself the care you need. Relate to yourself using **GIVE CARE**.
- Take your well-being seriously: The bigger the emotion, the more important it feels, the more you want to make sure you are not missing something important before deciding what to do.

TIP: Please be patient with yourself as you work to develop better relationships with your feelings; changing how you relate to your emotions and body sensations takes *lots* of practice.

Each effort you make (whether you notice or not!) helps toward your goal!

EXERCISES FOR TOPIC 22: HOW TO HELP YOUR FEELINGS HELP YOU

We hope you have been using your plan to keep yourself in your window of tolerance. We also hope you have been giving yourself lots of credit each time you notice the level of distress you are feeling and each time you practice healthy coping to help yourself stay within or get back into your window of tolerance.

We also hope you are working to collect safer experiences, doing the things that help you calm your alarm system (instead of things that get in the way of getting and feeling safer), and reducing your exposure to unhealthy and retraumatizing experiences.

In the information sheet for Topic 22, we talked about how to help your feelings help you. Please review the information sheet before continuing on to the exercises below. As with all work in this program, please make sure you are grounded before beginning this work. Go at a pace that is manageable for you, taking breaks to ground and use healthy coping as you need to.

Grounded? Let's start.

Written Exercises for Topic 22: How to Help Your Feelings Help You

If you have a difficult relationship with your feelings, you're not alone, and it's not your fault.

It can be very difficult for people who have experienced trauma to identify, accept, and safely experience their feelings and body sensations. Feeling too much or too little emotion (emotional feelings) and/or physical sensations (physical feelings) can lead people to not notice or to be overwhelmed by emotions and body cues. *Each of these difficulties is an understandable effect of having been traumatized. They are also important to work on as part of healing.*

Developing a healthy relationship with your feelings and body sensations is an important part of getting and feeling safer. A healthy relationship with your feelings can help you make good choices about how you want to live now. A healthy relationship with your body sensations can help you notice what your body needs to feel safe and healthy.

Being overwhelmed by or disconnected from bodily cues can lead people to eat and/or sleep too little or too much, or to not notice when they need medical care. Being overwhelmed by or disconnected from emotions can lead people to be more likely to be at risk or to engage in unhealthy or unsafe behaviors. So learning how to pay attention to and respond to body signals in healthy ways without getting overwhelmed can make a big difference toward helping you heal and protecting you from further trauma.

Written exercise 1: Identifying the levels of feelings and sensations that are comfortable for you

An important first step of this work is being aware of your level of comfort with different feelings and sensations. Why? Being aware of your level of comfort with different feelings and sensations can help you notice:

- Your range of tolerance for these different feelings and sensations—which can help you plan for how to keep yourself in your window of tolerance.
- Which feelings might be helpful and manageable to work on having better relationships with.

Below, we invite you to identify your level of comfort with different feelings and sensations. As you do this work, please put safety and healthy coping first. Pay attention to your level of distress and use your "Plan to keep myself in my window of tolerance" (from Topic 21) and healthy coping and safety plans as necessary.

Imagine that the lines below represent a range of feelings and sensations, from 0 (least intense) to 10 (feeling very intense feelings or sensations). What are the lowest and highest levels you feel comfortable having for each of the following feelings? Please circle the numbers that reflect the low and high ends of your window of tolerance.

Thirsty

| 0 | 1 | 2 | 3 | 4 | 5 | 6 | 7 | 8 | 9 | 10 |

(least intense)   *(most intense)*

Hungry

| 0 | 1 | 2 | 3 | 4 | 5 | 6 | 7 | 8 | 9 | 10 |

(least intense)   *(most intense)*

Full

| 0 | 1 | 2 | 3 | 4 | 5 | 6 | 7 | 8 | 9 | 10 |

(least intense)   *(most intense)*

Tired

| 0 | 1 | 2 | 3 | 4 | 5 | 6 | 7 | 8 | 9 | 10 |

(least intense)   *(most intense)*

Sick

| 0 | 1 | 2 | 3 | 4 | 5 | 6 | 7 | 8 | 9 | 10 |

(least intense) (most intense)*

Stressed/Tense

| 0 | 1 | 2 | 3 | 4 | 5 | 6 | 7 | 8 | 9 | 10 |

(least intense) (most intense)*

Afraid

| 0 | 1 | 2 | 3 | 4 | 5 | 6 | 7 | 8 | 9 | 10 |

(least intense) (most intense)*

Sad

| 0 | 1 | 2 | 3 | 4 | 5 | 6 | 7 | 8 | 9 | 10 |

(least intense) (most intense)*

Irritated/Mad

| 0 | 1 | 2 | 3 | 4 | 5 | 6 | 7 | 8 | 9 | 10 |

(least intense) (most intense)*

Surprised

| 0 | 1 | 2 | 3 | 4 | 5 | 6 | 7 | 8 | 9 | 10 |

(least intense) (most intense)*

Disgusted

| 0 | 1 | 2 | 3 | 4 | 5 | 6 | 7 | 8 | 9 | 10 |

(least intense) (most intense)*

Guilt

| 0 | 1 | 2 | 3 | 4 | 5 | 6 | 7 | 8 | 9 | 10 |

(least intense) (most intense)*

Shame

0	1	2	3	4	5	6	7	8	9	10

(least intense)   *(most intense)*

Happy/Glad

0	1	2	3	4	5	6	7	8	9	10

(least intense)   *(most intense)*

Interested

0	1	2	3	4	5	6	7	8	9	10

(least intense)   *(most intense)*

Connected to your body

0	1	2	3	4	5	6	7	8	9	10

(least intense)   *(most intense)*

Are you doing OK? Do you need a break to get grounded and practice healthy coping? If so, please do, and then come back.

Ready to continue?

Below, we talk about why people can have difficulty relating to their feelings, and we ask you to think about your current relationship to your feelings. As always, do this work at a pace that is manageable for you. Our goal is for you to get and feel safer—please put safety and healthy coping first. Pay attention to any early warning signs that might emerge, and follow your safety planning. If you start to feel overwhelmed or begin to dissociate, take a break, work on getting grounded, and practice healing-focused coping skills (things from your list of healthy things to do when feeling too much or too little that you began developing in Topic 3, and elaborated in your plan to keep yourself in your window of tolerance in Topic 21).

Written exercise 2: Your relationship with your feelings and sensations

Experiencing trauma (particularly as a child) can lead you to believe that feelings and bodily needs are bad or wrong. We learn how to deal with feelings by watching how the people around us deal with feelings when we are children. (If the people from your childhood handled their feelings safely and in healthy ways, you may have learned to do the same. If not, you may not have learned how to deal with feelings in healthy ways.) When people have experienced childhood trauma and family dysfunction, feelings and bodily needs can begin to seem dangerous.

When parents are healthy and know how to parent well, they recognize when a child is emotionally upset or needs to rest or eat. They reach out to the child and comfort them, and they may play with the child, read to them, feed them, encourage them to go to sleep, or engage in some other type of caring activity.

But when there are significant problems in a family, there may not be anyone who can help a child learn to take care of their emotions and their body's needs. This can make a child feel scared or ashamed of their body's needs and emotions. Trauma later in life can have similar effects.

Being scared or ashamed of bodily needs and emotions is an understandable result of very difficult circumstances. However, emotions are not bad or wrong, and neither are our bodies' physical needs.

Every child, teenager, and adult has a range of emotions and a range of basic physical needs. Every person has the right to be safe and comfortable and have their bodily needs met safely. Every person has the right to feel all their feelings and be curious about what their feelings are telling them. Our feelings are always there for a reason: to get our attention, to let us know that it feels like something important is happening.

If any of the difficulties we described above are true for you, we are hoping that you can begin to learn new ways of looking at feelings and bodily needs in these written and practice exercises. As always, your safety comes first: Take breaks if you need to, and follow your plan to keep yourself in your window of tolerance.

Are you grounded? If yes, continue.

Do any of your emotional feelings feel like they are "not allowed" or "not OK"?

_____

_____

_____

_____

_____

Do any of your bodily sensations feel like they are "not allowed" or "not OK"?

_____

_____

_____

_____

What do you do when you have emotions that feel like they are "not allowed" or "not OK"?

_____

_____

_____

_____

_____

What do you do when you have body sensations that feel like they are "not allowed" or "not OK"?

_____

_____

_____

_____

_____

Are there any people in your life who model healthy ways to cope with feelings and/or body sensations? What do you admire about the ways they deal with feelings or body sensations? How could _you_ use more of those ways of dealing with feelings?

_____

_____

_____

_____

_____

_____

Written exercise 3: Developing healthier guidelines for yourself

Some people seem to live by feelings and sensation "rules," such as "I must deny my feelings and not show them. I must not have any needs. I must meet other people's needs at all times. All body sensations are bad or dirty." These types of rules are unhealthy. They can contribute to people dissociating and/or engaging in risky, unhealthy, or unsafe behaviors.

As an adult, you have the power and right to make conscious choices, including about how to manage feelings and sensations. Perhaps you could create some healthier guidelines for yourself.

Here are some healthier guidelines to consider: "I am going to try to be aware of my needs and meet them in healthy ways. I am going to work hard to get a healthier relationship with my feelings and my body. I am healing, and I will learn to notice my feelings safely as I feel safe and ready to do so."

Can you use the space below to write guidelines that are healthy for you?

(This is a topic that can be helpful to talk about with your therapist. Because this can be a challenging topic, please remember to notice your level of distress and give yourself the care you need: Use grounding and take breaks as needed.)

If you have parts, and parts disagree about these topics, work with each other to understand your parts' underlying concerns—in other words, what is this part of me afraid will happen if I do this?—and determine how to address their concerns and do this work in a way that feels manageable. One option that can be helpful is allowing parts who are willing to start working with feelings in healthy ways to do so, while inviting parts who are not so sure about this to watch how this goes (if they'd like to!) from peaceful places. This process can be very challenging; if it is, we encourage you to talk to your therapist about how to negotiate and collaborate with your parts.

Healthier guidelines for responding to my emotions and physical sensations

---

_____

_____

_____

_____

_____

_____

If you have parts: Do different parts of you have different levels of awareness about your body and its healthy needs and messages? Do some parts feel feelings that other parts of you had to disconnect from (dissociate) to be able to make it through? If yes, consider how crucial these parts of you have been to your survival; by taking on those feelings for you, these parts helped you survive. In the space below, it might be helpful to acknowledge how helpful these parts were to you, and to think about how you can work together to give these parts the care they need and help them get their healthy needs met safely.

_____

_____

_____

_____

_____

_____

_____

_____

Practice Exercise for Topic 22: How to Help Your Feelings Help You

Please take some time each day to review the information sheet's suggestions about how to have a healthy relationship with your emotions and body sensations, and work to develop and follow new, healthier guidelines for your relationship with your feelings. Try to be aware of urges to follow old rules about feelings and your body. Be sure to give yourself lots of credit each time you notice this.

As you notice these urges, take these opportunities to try out your new guidelines as often as possible. Practice noticing the level of distress you are feeling and using healthy coping to help yourself stay within or get back into your window of tolerance. Be patient and compassionate with yourself. Lasting change takes practice and time. It is OK to go at a pace that is right for you. Keep at it!

Step by step, you will get there!

WHY NAMING FEELINGS CAN BE DIFFICULT

Information Sheet for Topic 23

Developing a healthy relationship with your emotions (feelings) is an important part of getting and feeling safer. Emotions help us notice when it feels like something important is happening and encourage us to do something that will help. A crucial part of improving your relationship with your emotions is learning how to name your feelings.

Why might emotions be difficult to name?

- People who experienced trauma often have difficulty identifying their feelings. Sometimes they can only recognize feeling bad or overwhelmed.
- Naming feelings can be particularly challenging for people who were made to feel that having emotions was not OK or who were never shown how emotions help or how to name what they were feeling.
- People who have difficulty identifying their feelings may be (unintentionally or intentionally) suppressing their feelings.

Why not just suppress my emotions?

- When you suppress feelings, you tend to lose touch with all emotions, not just the ones you do not want.
- If you are unable to feel emotions, you miss much of what makes life worth living. People without feelings may feel like their lives are empty.
- It is difficult (if not impossible) to enjoy life if you do not feel happiness, peacefulness, or pleasure. This is why it is so important to learn how to feel and tolerate all your feelings—so you can have a life with some pleasure and happiness, a life you can feel good about.

Due to trauma-based beliefs, the idea of feeling emotions (including happiness) may seem scary or wrong to some people. If you feel this way, review the signs that you might be having trauma-based thoughts, and work to shift these thoughts from trauma-based beliefs to healing-focused thinking. Work to change how you deal with your feelings at a pace that works for you.

TIP: Be patient, gentle, fair, and encouraging with yourself as you do this difficult but important work. Give yourself the care you need as you need it. Step by step, you'll get there!

EXERCISES FOR TOPIC 23: WHY NAMING FEELINGS CAN BE DIFFICULT

We hope you have been noticing urges to follow old rules about feelings and that you have been developing and reminding yourself of your new guidelines. We also hope you have been using your plan to keep yourself in your window of tolerance, giving yourself lots of credit each time you notice the level of distress you are feeling and practice healthy coping to help yourself stay in or get back into your window of tolerance.

In the information sheet for Topic 23, we talked about why naming feelings can be difficult and why not to suppress feelings. Please review the information sheet before continuing on to the exercises below.

As with all work in this program, make sure you are grounded before beginning this work. Go at a pace that is manageable for you, taking breaks to ground and use healthy coping as you need to.

Are you grounded? Let's start.

Written Exercise for Topic 23: Why Naming Feelings Can Be Difficult

A healthy relationship with your feelings is an important part of getting and feeling safer. Having a healthy relationship with your feelings can help you make good choices about how you want to live now—and can make your life feel richer and more rewarding.

An important step in this process is learning to notice and name your feelings when they first start to happen. It can be very difficult to do this important work, however. People who have experienced trauma often have difficulty identifying their feelings, and naming feelings can be particularly challenging for people who are used to dissociating or suppressing their feelings or who were never helped to name what they were feeling.

Knowing what our bodies are trying to tell us requires our curiosity and careful thinking. This is true of bodily sensations and emotions. We need to be curious about what the sensations in our bodies mean and to be thoughtful in trying to understand the physical signals our bodies give us. For example, it's not unusual to have difficulty knowing whether your body is trying to tell you that you're tired or hungry. Many people notice a feeling that feels like hunger (even when they've had enough to eat) when they start to get tired. The signals our bodies send us related to our emotional feelings can also be difficult to interpret, especially if you haven't been helped with this in the past. Doing this difficult but important work is easier if you can help yourself notice and remember your reasons for developing healthier relationships with your feelings.

Identifying your reasons for developing a healthier relationship with your feelings
If you have difficulty naming your feelings, find that you have a tendency to not feel your feelings or body signals, or alternate between not feeling your feelings or body signals and then feeling too much, review "Why not just suppress my emotions?" in Topic 23's information sheet (p. 190) and "Why might people want to work toward being more comfortable with having and recognizing their feelings and body sensations?" in Topic 22's information sheet (p. 179).

Then use the space below to write about the reasons that speak to you: What helps you want to begin to pay attention to and name your emotions? How would your life be better if you had a healthier relationship with your emotions and body sensations?

(*In addition to reviewing the information in this module, you may find it helpful to revisit what you wrote for Written exercise 2: Ways my life could be better if I were feeling safer in Topic 18 [p. 151]. If you have parts, please consider parts' answers and concerns about this. It can be helpful to talk to a therapist about this.*)

My reasons for developing healthier relationships with my feelings

_____

_____

_____

_____

_____

_____

_____

_____

_____

_____

_____

_____

_____

Practice Exercise for Topic 23: Why Naming Feelings Can Be Difficult

Continue working to be aware of urges to follow old rules about feelings and body sensations, and give yourself lots of credit each time you notice this. As you notice these urges, please take these opportunities to remind yourself as often as possible of the new guidelines you've been developing for yourself. Practice noticing the level of distress you are feeling and using healthy coping to help yourself stay in or get back into your window of tolerance.

We also encourage you to spend a little time each day reminding yourself of *your* reasons to develop a healthier relationship with your emotions and body sensations, adding to the list as you notice more reasons to do this important work.

Don't forget to notice and give yourself credit for each bit of progress—each step you take makes a difference in helping your brain (and all of who you are) heal.

Be compassionate with yourself as you practice—step by step, you will get there!

NAMING FEELINGS

Information Sheet for Topic 24

Emotions help us notice when it feels like something important is happening, and they encourage us to do something that will help us. Learning how to recognize and name your feelings makes it easier for your feelings to be helpful instead of confusing and upsetting.

What can help me name my feelings?

Paying attention to your body sensations helps you know what you are feeling.[1]

Basic feeling	Related feelings	Related sensations	What this feeling tries to help you notice
Sad	Grief, feeling down, discouraged, depressed	Heaviness; aching, especially around the heart; tightness or soreness in the throat	Feeling that you have lost, are losing, or will lose someone or something important to you
Glad	Happy, joy, pleased, confident	Lightness in the body, energetic, heart feels free and light	Feeling that something good has happened, is happening, or will happen
Mad	Annoyed, irritated, frustrated, angry, enraged	Tightness in the chest, neck, and/or shoulders; tension in the hands or jaw; heart beating quickly; breathing is fast and intense	Feeling that something not fair, not right, and/or not OK has happened, is happening, or will happen
Afraid	Nervous, anxious, fearful, scared, terrified	Heart beating quickly, breathing is rapid and shallow; stomach and intestines feel "knotted," tense, unsettled, nauseous; sweaty; clammy and cold; want to escape	Feeling that something threatening has happened, is happening, or will happen

---

[1] Informed in part by Tomkins, 1962, 1963, 1991.

Basic feeling	Related feelings	Related sensations	What this feeling tries to help you notice
Interested	Attentive, focused, excited	Alert, heart beating quickly, eyes focused on what is interesting	Feeling that something interesting has happened, is happening, or will happen
Surprised	Taken aback, startled, shocked	Alert, on guard, heart beating quickly, "wide eyes"	Feeling that something unanticipated has happened, is happening, or will happen
Shame	Embarrassed, humiliated, feeling bad about self	Head drops to hide face; face is flushed and hot; sweaty; want to disappear and hide	Feeling that you are (and are seen by others as) "bad," have been seen as "bad," or will be seen as "bad"
Guilt	Feeling bad about something you've done, wishing you hadn't done something	Stomach and intestines feel tense, unsettled	Feeling that you've done something you wish you hadn't; feeling that you want to undo, take back, or repair something you've done
Disgust	Revolted, "grossed out"	Nose wrinkling as if smelling something spoiled, frowning, pulling away	Feeling that something is, will be, or has been "sickening"

EXERCISES FOR TOPIC 24: NAMING FEELINGS

We hope you have been noticing urges to follow old rules about feelings, reminding yourself of your new guidelines, and spending a little time each day reminding yourself of your reasons to have a better relationship with your feelings, adding to the list as you notice more reasons to do this important work. We also hope you have been using your plan to keep yourself in your window of tolerance, giving yourself lots of credit each time you notice the level of distress you are feeling and practicing healthy coping to help yourself stay in or get back into your window of tolerance.

In the information sheet for Topic 24, we talked about naming feelings. Please review this information before continuing on to the exercises below.

As with all work in this program, make sure you are grounded before beginning this work. Go at a pace that is manageable for you, taking breaks to ground and use healthy coping as you need to.

Are you grounded? Let's start.

Written Exercise for Topic 24: Naming Feelings

Preparing to practice paying attention to and naming feelings
It can be very difficult for people who have experienced trauma to identify, accept, and safely experience their feelings. At the same time, it is also true that developing a healthy relationship with your feelings is an important part of getting and feeling safer: A healthy relationship with your feelings can help you make good choices about how you want to live now.

The first and most important step in learning to pay attention to and name feelings is to develop a plan for doing this work that you feel good about.

For example: Consider starting with brief practice sessions—maybe just a few seconds, and definitely less than a minute! As you get better at tolerating feelings, you can extend the time. Some people find it helps to set a timer so they do not lose track of time and feel more in control while practicing tolerating feelings.

In the series of questions below, we encourage you to think about how to help yourself do this work.

1. Which feeling or body sensation that you would like to "widen your window of tolerance" for (be better able to tolerate) is easiest for you to experience?

2. What length of time feels manageable to start with?

(We recommend that you start by allowing yourself to feel that feeling for a very brief period of time—maybe just a few seconds! After that is manageable, maybe you could extend the time by small increments.)

_____

3. What healthy ways of helping yourself could help make this feel manageable?

(What skills or recommendations from this program could help? Consider using a before, during, and after plan [see Topic 12, p. 97] or dial imagery [see Topic 7, p. 55] to dial down overwhelming feelings. Or, if you're working toward improving your relationship with body sensations, start with paying attention to one tiny "OK" area of your body, such as your forehead or the tip of a pinky. If some feelings are really challenging, consider practicing tolerating those feelings when you are with your therapist.)

Please use the space below to write about how you *specifically* would like to do this work.

_____

_____

_____

_____

_____

_____

_____

_____

_____

_____

_____

_____

_____

_____

_____

_____

_____

_____

_____

_____

_____

If you have parts, it is important to do feelings work in a way that is tolerable for all parts of you. We are not suggesting that all parts should work on tolerating all feelings at once. Instead, you might consider which parts are ready to work on noticing a feeling, focusing on one feeling at a time. Some parts may not be ready to work on tolerating and naming feelings; if so, please think about how you might protect those parts.

(For example, do all parts have a peaceful place inside that they can go to so that they do not have to have feelings they do not yet feel ready for? If not, consider developing peaceful place imagery.)

Please use the space below to work with parts to help them understand why this is important for all of you. Be curious about what they think, and take any concerns they have seriously. Find ways to help make this work manageable for parts so that they can genuinely agree that it is OK to practice identifying feelings. Remember that going slower will help you get there faster. You may wish to talk about this in therapy.

_____

_____

_____

_____

_____

_____

_____

_____

_____

_____

_____

_____

_____

_____

Practice Exercise for Topic 24: Naming Feelings

Continue working to be aware of urges to follow old rules about feelings. Please take these opportunities to remind yourself of your new feelings guidelines (Topic 22, p. 187) and your reasons for developing a healthier relationship with your feelings (Topic 23, p. 193). Practice noticing the level of distress you are feeling and using healthy coping to help yourself stay in (or get back into) your window of tolerance by following your plan (Topic 21, p. 175).

If you (and all parts, if you have parts) have a plan to practice noticing and naming feelings, please follow that plan. If you haven't finished developing that plan yet, take a little time each day to work on creating a plan to practice noticing and naming feelings that feels manageable.

Be patient and compassionate with yourself as you do this difficult and important work. Remember that it is OK to go at a pace that is right for you and that lasting change takes practice and time. Keep at it—and keep giving yourself credit for all the work you are doing!

Step by step, you will get there!

References for Topic 24

Tomkins, S. S. (1962). *Affect imagery consciousness: Vol. I. The positive affects.* Springer.
Tomkins, S. S. (1963). *Affect imagery consciousness: Vol. II. The negative affects.* Springer.
Tomkins, S. S. (1991). *Affect imagery consciousness: Vol. III. The negative affects: Anger and fear.* Springer.

SELF-UNDERSTANDING THROUGH COMPASSION: ACCEPTING ALL YOUR FEELINGS

Information Sheet for Topic 25

Emotions (feelings) help us notice when it feels like something important is happening, and they encourage us to do something that will help improve the situation. Developing a healthy relationship with your emotions is an important part of the process of getting and feeling safer. For people with dissociative parts/voices, this involves working with the parts/voices to understand their concerns and learn how to collaborate toward getting healthy needs met safely.

What does accepting your feelings (and parts) mean?

- Recognizing and acknowledging when you are (or part of you is) having a feeling, even if you do not like having it. ("I'm having this feeling right now.")
- Assuming that the feeling makes sense given your past, what is happening, or what you're worrying might happen, and having compassion with yourself for the feeling.
- Being curious about whether you're missing something, what is best for you in the here and now, and making sure you are grounded before making decisions.
- Using healthy coping skills to manage difficult feelings (follow your healthy coping and safety plans).

Later, when you are grounded and it is manageable, allow yourself to be curious about how the feeling makes sense given your past, and express empathy to yourself. (Note: This last step is easiest when you are in your window of tolerance. You may need the help of your therapist to develop compassion for all your feelings/parts. Staying safe should continue to be your top priority.)

What does accepting your feelings (and parts) not mean?

- "Going along with" unhealthy impulses connected with a feeling.
- That you have to "be OK with" having a particular feeling or impulse.

Important information for people with dissociative parts/voices

- Dissociative parts/voices develop to help you survive.
- All parts have strengths, even if you cannot recognize their strengths yet.
- Learning how parts have been helpful during difficult times may help you begin to understand your parts. That can help parts learn to cooperate.
- Beginning to respect how parts think and feel is an important step in healing.
- Respecting different parts does not mean that you have to agree with everything they think and want to do. Instead, it means learning to ease up on inside "wars" and conflicts and working to understand parts' concerns and respectfully collaborate toward getting healthy needs met safely.
- In stressful situations, parts may have different trauma-related reactions.
- Some parts may still think the present IS the past. To help those parts, it is **very** important to help them get oriented to and anchored in the present moment.

How can I develop a healthy relationship with my emotions (and parts)?

Work toward relating to yourself with curiosity and compassion. Relate to your emotions (and parts, if you have them) with curiosity. Ask yourself:

- What am I (my parts) feeling, and why might I (my parts) be feeling this way?
- Is there something I am missing? (Am I grounded/connected to the here and now?)
- Are there things I am not paying attention to? Am I being fair?
- What can I do that will best help me toward having the life I want?

Relate to yourself with compassion:

- Remind yourself that feelings always make sense based on what we *think* is happening/has happened/might happen.
- Remember, it is difficult to notice (and easy to minimize) things that do not fit what you are thinking and feeling. Give yourself lots of credit if you can notice something you had not noticed before!
- Give yourself the care you need. Relate to yourself using **GIVE CARE**.
- Take your well-being seriously: The bigger the emotion, the more important it feels, the more you want to make sure you are not missing something important before deciding what to do.

EXERCISES FOR TOPIC 25: SELF-UNDERSTANDING THROUGH COMPASSION: ACCEPTING ALL YOUR FEELINGS

We hope you have been noticing urges to follow old rules about feelings, reminding yourself of your new feelings guidelines as often as possible, and reminding yourself of your reasons to work toward healthier relationships with your feelings. We also hope you have been working toward noticing and naming feelings safely, using your plan to keep yourself in your window of tolerance, and giving yourself lots of credit for all the work you are doing to help yourself heal.

In the information sheet for Topic 25, we talked about relating to your feelings (and parts, if you have parts) with self-compassion and curiosity. Please review the information sheet before continuing on. As with all work in this program, make sure you are grounded before beginning this work. Go at a pace that is manageable for you, taking breaks to ground and use healthy coping as you need to.

Are you grounded? Let's start.

Written Exercise for Topic 25: Self-Understanding Through Compassion: Accepting All Your Feelings

Accepting your feelings and needs

Many people who have experienced trauma feel shame for having trauma-related feelings and/ or reactions, but this is not fair. Trauma-related feelings, reactions, and symptoms are normal for people who have experienced trauma. When people feel uncomfortable or ashamed of feelings or experiences, they may push them away (suppress them) or dissociate them. This can lead to these feelings/experiences coming back at an intense level and feeling too much all at once, making it difficult to help yourself manage these intense emotions in healthy ways. For people who have parts, dissociating emotions or other experiences can also contribute to feeling fragmented, with dissociative parts that feel disconnected or separate. Please don't shame yourself about any of these trauma-related difficulties—and please know that, with practice, things can be different.

You have a right to all of your feelings. You have a right to self-compassion and to take good care of yourself. All your feelings and parts (if you have parts) are there for a reason.

Although it may not always feel like it, all of your feelings are there to help you, and all of your feelings are important. Each of your feelings is there to get your attention (to let you know that it feels like something important is happening) and to get you curious about what is happening and what could help improve the situation.

If you have parts, all parts of you are important. All of who you are deserves self-compassion. All parts deserve to be safe and to be treated kindly and with respect. Approach your parts with curiosity and a willingness to understand those sides of yourself.

Self-compassion is difficult for many people; the good news is that it gets easier (and things get better) if you allow yourself to increasingly approach yourself (and parts) with the same kind, compassionate curiosity you would show to someone you deeply care about. Ask yourself compassionately:

- "How am I doing?"
- "What are my concerns?"
- "What do I need?" (GIVE CARE to yourself.)
- "Is there something I'm not noticing or not paying attention to that would lead me to feel differently or help me handle the situation better?"
- "Which of my options is most likely to help me build the kind of life I want for myself?"

Keep reminding yourself that your reactions make sense given what you think is happening, even if your reactions don't always fit the here and now—and that you are taking steps to help yourself heal from being at heightened risk for intrusive trauma-related emotions, reactions, and symptoms.

Although this practice can be difficult at first, you will keep making progress on this—and it will slowly get easier—as you keep working on it. You might notice that approaching yourself with compassion and respect makes things more manageable and reduces some of the shame you may feel.

The exercises for this topic focus on increasing self-compassion and self-understanding in relation to your feelings and needs. If you find yourself feeling stuck, consider whether you might be having trauma-based thoughts, and work to address them (see Topic 17). (Note: The questions in this topic's written exercise can be good to talk about with your therapist.) As always, your safety comes first: Pay attention to your level of distress, take breaks and use skills if you need to, and follow your healthy coping and safety plans.

Do you have difficulty accepting your feelings or needs? If yes, which?

(If you have parts, please write about which feelings are difficult for them, too. You may wish to share this list with your therapist.)

_____

_____

_____

_____

_____

_____

Can you imagine situations where those feelings or needs make sense? Have you seen people manage those feelings or needs safely and effectively? If yes, how might you help yourself do things in those ways? (You may also find it helpful to review previous modules for suggestions—and this is a good topic to ask your therapist for help with if you find yourself getting stuck.)

_____

_____

_____

_____

_____

_____

_____

_____

_____

_____

_____

_____

_____

For people who have parts, please approach the next questions with curiosity and compassion: All parts deserve to be safe and to be treated kindly and respectfully.

Do you have difficulty accepting parts of yourself? Are you aware of (or can you imagine) how those parts have helped you? Could you invite the parts you are having difficulty with to help you understand their underlying concerns—in other words, what are they trying to avoid? (Please do this without sharing any overwhelming memories—and, if necessary, consider sharing information at a "headline" level [i.e., using a couple of words to summarize, like a newspaper headline].)

If there are parts you disagree with about behaviors they do or want to do, could you work together to find goals you share? Or ways of doing things that are OK for all parts of you? (Look for healthy compromises that respect the concerns of all involved.) This is another good topic to ask your therapist for help with if you find yourself getting stuck.

_____

_____

_____

_____

_____

_____

_____

_____

_____

_____

_____

_____

_____

_____

_____

_____

_____

_____

_____

_____

_____

Practice Exercise for Topic 25: Self-Understanding Through Compassion: Accepting All Your Feelings

We encourage you to practice self-compassion in relation to your feelings and needs. Practice following the suggestions in the information sheet section "How can I develop a healthy relationship with my emotions (and parts)?" (p. 201). Check in with yourself (and your parts, if you have parts) regularly, asking yourself compassionately:

- "How am I doing?"
- "Are there things I'm not noticing or not paying attention to?"
- "What would help?"

If you start to feel impatient with yourself, remind yourself that your reactions make sense given the experiences you have had and what it feels like is happening. What would you tell a child who described the same situation? Would you be critical of a child who felt scared, ashamed, or humiliated or who needed reassurance that they were safe or cared for?

See if you can talk to yourself as kindly as you would to a child who you love. You can learn to talk to yourself in the same kind way. Give yourself the care you need with **GIVE CARE** (see Topic 10 on p. 75). It is especially important to learn to do kind, reassuring self-talk when you feel young, or ashamed, or vulnerable, or afraid. You could learn to say something like, "You are safe now. It's going to be OK."

If you talk compassionately to yourself and give yourself (and your parts, if you have parts) the care you need, it may help all of who you are stay oriented to the present. It may help you to not slip back into past painful memories.

We would also like you to keep practicing healthy coping skills to stay within your window of tolerance. Don't expect perfection. This takes time. Give yourself credit for doing this difficult work!

Step by step, you'll get there!

SAFELY PRACTICING NOTICING AND NAMING FEELINGS

Information Sheet for Topic 26

Developing a healthy relationship with your emotions is an important part of the process of getting and feeling safer. Emotions help us notice when it feels like something important is happening, and they encourage us to do something that will help us. To build a healthy relationship with your emotions and learn how to tolerate feelings in healthy ways, practice having feelings safely.

What is a good approach to practice noticing and naming feelings?

- **Go at a pace that is right for you.** When practicing, try to take what feels like a manageable next step. Remind yourself to be patient and self-compassionate. Lasting change takes practice and time! Use healthy coping skills (such as grounding, deep breathing, and "feelings dial" regulators) if you start to feel too much or too little.

- **If you have parts, work to help them understand why this is important for all of you.** Listen to and take any concerns they have seriously. Find ways to help make this work manageable for your parts so that they can genuinely agree that it is OK to practice identifying feelings.

- **Make early practice sessions brief** (less than a minute!), extending the length of time as you get more comfortable.

Reminder: To develop healthy relationships with emotions (and parts)

Work toward relating to all parts of yourself with curiosity and compassion.

Ask yourself: What am I (my parts) feeling? Why might I (my parts) be feeling this way? Is there something I am missing? Are there things I am not paying attention to? Am I being fair? What can I do that will best help address the situation?

Remind yourself: Feelings always make sense based on what we think is happening/has happened/will happen. It is difficult to notice (and easy to minimize) things that do not fit what you are feeling. Give yourself lots of credit if you can notice something you had not noticed before! Give yourself the care you need.

TIP: Be curious about what is best for you in the here and now, with the strengths and resources you have now as an adult. The bigger the emotion, the more important it feels, the more you want to make sure you are not missing something important before deciding what to do.

What are the steps to practice noticing and naming feelings?

1. **Get grounded.** Orient yourself to and anchor yourself in the present before you begin to practice.

2. **Tune in to yourself.** Do you notice any feelings? Sometimes feelings are small; sometimes they are bigger. Sometimes they seem close by, and sometimes they seem further away. Take a moment and notice if you feel anything.

3. If you notice a feeling, **focus your attention on that feeling**. Recognize having the feeling. That is, allow yourself to admit that you are having the feeling, whether or not you like having it. Remind yourself that feelings pass and that you are taking this brief time to practice feeling what you are feeling. You may not notice feeling something during the time you have set aside to practice noticing feelings. That's OK—just keep making time to practice safely, and you will get there!

4. If you are aware of a feeling, **notice where you feel it**: Do you feel it in a particular place in your body? (To do this, you may need to work on grounding and staying connected to being safe in the present day and time.)

5. You may notice having different feelings at the same time—this is not unusual. (If having too many feelings at the same time is overwhelming, **see if you can focus in on the most manageable feeling for a brief period of time.**)

6. **Try to identify what you are feeling.** Remember: The basic feelings are sad, glad, mad, afraid, interested, surprised, shame, guilt, and disgust. It is OK if you are not sure what you are feeling. Just notice whatever you experience.

7. **If you are not sure which feeling you are having, think of times you felt similarly to see if you can match this feeling with how you were feeling then.** Again, it is OK if this is difficult. Be patient with yourself. You are trying to teach your brain to do things that it may have been avoiding for years. It will take time to learn to respond to feelings in a new way. Be encouraging to yourself and keep trying. Take breaks. Use healthy coping if you need to.

8. **Give yourself lots of credit for having taken time to notice and name your feelings!** This is a very important part of your healing process. You are helping your brain heal and make new connections each time you practice!

EXERCISES FOR TOPIC 26: SAFELY PRACTICING NOTICING AND NAMING FEELINGS

We hope you have been noticing urges to follow old rules about feelings, reminding yourself of your new feelings guidelines and your reasons to work toward healthier, self-compassionate relationships with your feelings. We also hope you have been working toward noticing and naming feelings safely and using your plan to keep yourself in your window of tolerance, giving yourself lots of credit each time you notice your level of distress and practice healthy coping to help yourself stay in or get back into your window of tolerance.

In the information sheet for Topic 26, we talked about how to safely practice naming feelings. Please review the information sheet before continuing on to the exercises below.

As with all work in this program, make sure you are grounded before beginning this work. Go at a pace that is manageable for you, taking breaks to ground and use healthy coping as you need to.

Are you grounded? Let's start.

Written Exercise for Topic 26: Safely Practicing Noticing and Naming Feelings

What has helped/might help in manageably paying attention to feelings?
You may have already given yourself permission to practice paying attention to and naming your feelings for limited periods of time. If you were able to do this, give yourself credit for taking this healthy but often difficult step. Use the space below to describe what it feels like to be learning how to pay attention to yourself and your feelings, what worked well, and what is still difficult. Work to have compassion with yourself—this is a process that will take time.

If you have not yet been ready to begin practicing paying attention to and naming your feelings, that is OK—we want you to go at a pace that works for you! Building on the work you have been doing over the "feelings" exercises in this module, use the space below to identify healthy ways of helping this (i.e., practicing paying attention to and naming your feelings) feel manageable. As you do, feel free to review previous modules to help yourself select skills or remind yourself of recommendations that you feel could be of help.

(**Once again: If you have parts**, it is important to do this work in a way that is tolerable for all parts of you. Please also use the space below to think about this work with parts. Be curious about what they think, and take any concerns they have seriously. Find ways to help make this work manageable for all parts so that you can all genuinely agree that it is OK to practice identifying feelings. You may wish to talk about this in therapy.)

_____

_____

_____

_____

_____

_____

_____

_____

_____

_____

_____

_____

_____

_____

_____

Practice Exercise for Topic 26: Safely Practicing Noticing and Naming Feelings

Continue working to be aware of urges to follow old rules about feelings. Give yourself lots of credit each time you notice these urges, and remind yourself of your new feelings guidelines (see Topic 22) and reasons to develop healthier relationships with your feelings (see Topic 24). Practice noticing the level of distress you are feeling (see Topic 21), and use healthy coping to help yourself stay in or get back into your window of tolerance.

Once you (and all parts, if you have parts) have a plan for beginning to practice noticing and naming feelings, please follow the **steps for practicing noticing and naming feelings** described in the information sheet for Topic 26.

Again, it is normal for this to be difficult. Please be patient with yourself. You are trying to teach your brain to do things that it may have been avoiding for years. It will take time to learn to respond to feelings in a new way. Be encouraging to yourself and keep trying. Take breaks, and give yourself the care you need, including healthy coping if you need to.

When you do this work, **please give yourself lots of credit for practicing noticing and naming your feelings**! This is a very important part of your healing process. You are helping your brain heal and make new connections each time you practice!

Be patient and compassionate with yourself. Lasting change takes practice and time. It is OK to go at a pace that is right for you. Keep at it.

Step by step, you will get there!

GUILT, SHAME, AND SELF-COMPASSION

Information Sheet for Topic 27

People who have experienced trauma are often caught in a struggle with guilt and shame. These feelings can come from believing untrue, harsh things that were said to them. They may unfairly blame themselves for traumas they experienced. They may take on guilt and shame that actually belong to the person(s) who hurt them. Trauma-based beliefs make these feelings *feel* fair even though they are NOT fair. Please work to notice unfair, untrue trauma-based beliefs, and replace them with compassionate, healing-focused thoughts.

What is guilt?

Guilt involves feeling bad and regretful about things you have done (or for *not* doing something).

Guilt motivates you to do things that help you live your life in a way that is consistent with your values.

Thoughts that accompany guilt can be something like, "I cannot believe I did that; that is not the way I want to be." When feeling guilt, you may notice wanting to find some way to make amends and/or to take steps to do things differently in the future.

What is shame?

Shame involves feeling like an unworthy or bad person. Shame often makes people want to hide, "disappear," or not be seen. Sometimes a person experiences some shame alongside guilt, but shame tends to fade as the person shifts toward making amends and doing things differently. If shame persists, it can become toxic and debilitating.

Shame can trigger impulses to avoid feelings, withdraw from others, or harshly criticize or be aggressive toward oneself or others. Shame can trigger strong urges to engage in unhealthy behaviors. Toxic shame makes people believe that they do not deserve compassion or to get their needs met safely.

Thoughts that can accompany toxic shame include "I am bad and wrong," "I do not deserve good things," or even "I deserve bad things to happen to me."

How can I determine if I am being unfair with myself?

If you feel bad (guilty) about something you have done, you cannot be an all-bad person: "All-bad" people do not feel bad about what they do. Instead of being harsh with yourself, give yourself the care you need to help yourself do things differently in the future.

Differences between healthy guilt and toxic shame

Toxic shame	Healthy guilt
Underlying thought: • "*I* am bad and wrong" (because of what I did/what happened).	Underlying thought: • "I feel bad about what I've *done*."
Is a trauma-related <u>symptom of depression</u> that: • Keeps you stuck in a pattern of harsh self-criticism/beating yourself up • Saps the energy you have • Leaves you feeling helpless/hopeless • Can lead to an unfair, untrue belief that you don't deserve good things to happen (or worse, that you deserve bad things to happen) • Leaves you without the energy you need to do the hard work involved in making changes, making change difficult	Is an emotion (related to sadness) that: • Motivates you to understand what happened and how to do things differently in the future • Gives you energy to make the changes you need to make to improve the future/forgive yourself
Is maintained by harsh self-criticism and trauma-based thoughts and beliefs	Is made possible by healthy self-compassion (Give yourself the care you need to make changes that will improve the future. Use GIVE CARE.)
Puts you at risk of making more mistakes	Helps you make changes that will improve the future

How can I help myself get out of toxic shame?

1. Learn to recognize the signs of toxic shame *(see above)* and shaming thoughts.
2. Remind yourself that it is not fair to think of yourself as "bad" if you feel bad about something you've done ("bad" people don't feel bad about the things they do).
3. If you feel bad about something you've done, instead of harshly criticizing and shaming yourself, give yourself the care you need to help yourself understand how the events happened and how to prevent similar mistakes in the future.

EXERCISES FOR TOPIC 27: GUILT, SHAME, AND SELF-COMPASSION

We hope you have been reminding yourself of your new feelings guidelines and your reasons to work toward a healthier, self-compassionate relationship with your feelings and all of who you are. We also hope you have been working toward noticing and naming feelings safely and using your plan to keep yourself in your window of tolerance, giving yourself lots of credit for all the work you are doing to help yourself heal.

In the information sheet for Topic 27, we talked about guilt, shame, and self-compassion. Please review the information sheet before continuing on. As with all work in this program, make sure you are grounded before beginning this work. Go at a pace that is manageable for you, checking in with yourself periodically to notice your level of distress, and taking breaks to ground and give yourself the care you need as you need to.

Grounded? Let's start.

Written Exercises for Topic 27: Guilt, Shame, and Self-Compassion

Many people who have experienced trauma feel unfair shame and guilt due to trauma-based thoughts. Trauma-based thoughts make these feelings *feel* fair even though they are NOT fair.

Working to increase self-compassion and reduce shame, guilt, and trauma-based thoughts is crucial to healing. As you work on these topics, please take extra care to use the skills you have been practicing to stay grounded and manage emotions safely. Remember to go at a pace that works for you.

Written exercise 1: Recognizing shame and shaming thoughts
When people feel shame, they may look down or have difficulty looking others in the eye. They may feel a strong desire to not be seen or truly known. Their faces may also get flushed and hot, and it can be difficult to think clearly. Shame is usually triggered by shaming thoughts. Shame can lead to very distorted views about yourself and others.

You have been working on shaming thoughts in different ways throughout this program. We hope this work has begun to help reduce the power of some of these beliefs, but we also know that changing these old beliefs can take a long time.

The table that follows presents some recovery-focused compassionate responses to shame-based thoughts.[2] (You may recognize some of these from earlier exercises; we include them here to make it easier for you to access and use them.)

As you go through the table, make a mark next to any of the "shaming thoughts" examples that you tell yourself, and circle example "recovery-focused, self-compassionate thoughts" that you could remind yourself of instead.

---

[2] Informed by Boon, Steele, and van der Hart, 2011, pp. 232–235; Najavits, 2002, p. 216; Williams & Poijula, 2002, p. 117.

Shaming thoughts *(Trauma-based thoughts make these thoughts feel fair even though they are NOT fair.)*	Recovery-focused, self-compassionate thoughts *(These thoughts are more fair and healthy.)*
"I'm no good." "I'm bad." "I'm weak."	"I have difficulties from being hurt, but having been hurt does not make me bad." "I have strengths and weaknesses, like everyone. I am working toward healing and making improvements in my life."
"I don't deserve help." "Others deserve good things more than I do."	"I deserve help and healing, just like all people deserve help and healing." "I do not have to be perfect to be OK, worthy of care, or deserving of safety."
"What I need does not matter."	"Everyone's needs matter, including mine."
"I deserve to be treated poorly."	"I deserve to get my needs met safely. It is OK and healthy to expect respect and to not stay in situations where I am being disrespected."
"I do not deserve to speak up for myself or ask for things."	"To build healthy relationships, it is important to express my needs and say when I do not like or do not want something. It is healthy and strong to be able to say 'no' to people if what they want is not good for me. If I begin to feel it is not OK to say 'no' in a relationship, it is time to pay close attention to the relationship. I need to think about whether the person is healthy for me. If I am concerned that I may be in an unsafe or unhealthy relationship, I will protect myself and talk to my therapist."

Notice that *recovery-focused thoughts do not ignore difficulties or negative information.* Instead, they tend to incorporate *more* information, including *context, positives,* and *strengths. Self-compassionate, fair thoughts acknowledge the realities of the present and promote healing.*

Written exercise 2: Noticing how you respond to shame
Shame can feel really toxic. It can easily become overwhelming. With practice, you can learn to respond to shame with self-compassion that challenges unfair thoughts and helps you engage in self-care.

When people are unable to challenge shaming beliefs, however, they tend to act in ways that perpetuate their shame. People who experience intense shame tend to respond by avoiding their feelings, withdrawing from others, and/or harshly criticizing (or punishing) themselves or others.[3]

Doing these shame-driven things ("following shame scripts") makes it difficult to heal. Acting as if the shaming thoughts are true reinforces the untrue belief that the shame is deserved.

---

[3] Nathanson, 1992.

In the exercise below, consider your responses when you feel shame. As you do, please practice looking at yourself with self-compassion. Talk to yourself as you would talk to someone who is hurting and deserves kindness as they make changes that will reduce their pain.

1. In which situations do you tend to avoid your feelings?

_____

_____

_____

_____

_____

_____

_____

2. In which situations do you tend to withdraw from others?

_____

_____

_____

_____

_____

_____

_____

3. In which situations do you tend to harshly criticize (or punish) yourself?

_____

_____

_____

_____

_____

_____

4. Are there any situations where you tend to harshly criticize (or punish) others?

_____

_____

_____

_____

_____

_____

Written exercise 3: Shifting from shaming thoughts to recovery-focused, self-compassionate thoughts

For each situation you listed in the four questions above, see if you can find a shaming thought that creates your feelings and behaviors. List it in the "Shaming thoughts/situation" column in the table below. Then see if you can identify self-compassionate thoughts and behaviors (e.g., skills you have been learning as part of this program) that you can practice instead. Add those to the "Self-compassionate thoughts and behaviors" column.

(As you do this work, you may find it helpful to review Topics 10, 11, and 17 and the recovery-focused, self-compassionate thought examples above [p. 217]. Remember to take this work at a pace that is manageable for you. If you find yourself having difficulty completing this exercise, consider talking to your therapist about this.)

Shaming thoughts/situation	Self-compassionate thoughts and behaviors

Practice Exercise for Topic 27: Guilt, Shame, and Self-Compassion

We encourage you to practice changing your responses to shame. Practice using the self-compassionate thoughts and behaviors you identified as part of the Written Exercise 3, including (and especially) when you are beginning to feel shame, have shame-based thoughts, or feel a pull to follow shame scripts.

Be patient and compassionate with yourself as you do this work. Make sure to give yourself credit for making progress when you are able to:

1. Notice you are feeling shame
2. Notice that trauma-based thoughts are perpetuating the shame
3. Respond to/challenge shaming thoughts with self-compassionate thoughts
4. Practice self-compassionate thoughts and behaviors when you find yourself wanting to do shame-perpetuating behaviors (i.e., avoiding, withdrawing, or being harsh with yourself or others).

Each of these actions represents a meaningful step toward helping yourself shift away from trauma-based shaming thoughts and toward recovery- and healing-focused thinking. Replacing shaming thoughts and shame scripts with self-compassionate thoughts and behaviors takes effort and lots of practice. Give yourself credit for doing this difficult work! You can feel proud about working hard to heal. Be patient with yourself. Lasting change takes practice and time. Keep at it—step by step, you'll get there!

REMEMBER:

As you continue through the program, strive to integrate what you've been learning into your daily routines. We recognize that this is much easier said than done, so please be patient with yourself as you work toward getting better and better at:

- getting your healthy needs met safely
- noticing where you are in your window of tolerance
- grounding
- separating past from present
- planning for difficult situations
- recognizing early warning signs
- giving yourself the care you need to manage difficult situations, break the cycle of unhealthy behavior, reduce trauma-related reactions, and heal trauma's impact on the brain
- recognizing and addressing trauma-based thoughts
- improving your relationship with your emotions and all of who you are
- recognizing shaming thoughts and shame-driven behaviors and replacing them with self-compassionate thoughts and behaviors
- noticing and giving yourself credit for progress.

Congratulations on completing the seventh module! Step by step, you're getting there!

In the next module, we'll offer additional information and exercises to help you continue to build on all the work you've been doing to get and feel safer.

References for Topic 27

Boon, S., Steele, K., & van der Hart, O. (2011). *Coping with trauma-related dissociation: Skills training for patients.* W. W. Norton & Company.

Najavits, L. M. (2002). *Seeking safety: A treatment manual for PTSD and substance abuse.* Guilford Press.

Nathanson, D.L. (1992). *Shame and pride: Affect, sex, and the birth of the self.* Norton.

Williams, M. B., & Poijula, S. (2002). *The PTSD workbook: Simple, effective techniques for overcoming traumatic stress symptoms.* New Harbinger Publications.

MODULE 8

Sticking With the Process and Building on Progress

Over the course of this program, you've been learning:

- About common trauma-related symptoms and impacts on people's feelings, relationships, and views about themselves and the world
- How to help yourself (including your brain) heal from the effects of trauma, starting with healthy ways to manage trauma-related symptoms, including experiences of feeling too much or too little
- How to have healthy relationships, starting with your relationships with yourself—with all of your emotions and all of who you are—including increasing self-compassion, getting your healthy needs met safely, and giving yourself the care you need.

To help you put what you've been learning into practice, you've been completing written and practice exercises. You have hopefully also been giving yourself credit for your all your hard work and noticing improvements as you go! (And if you haven't yet, this is a good time to do so!)

This module will help you learn:

- how to keep making progress toward feeling safer—including feeling safe while feeling your feelings
- how to help yourself to feel good
- how to keep healing.

This module will help you practice:

- noticing and giving yourself credit for what you have been doing and what is working well
- identifying and addressing factors that may be keeping you from feeling safer and better
- recognizing the changes you've made, what has helped, and what you'd like to practice more.

This module invites you to bring together all you've been practicing as part of this program to help you continue to make progress toward getting and feeling safer. Please give yourself the care you need as you do this work.

FEELING SAFE TAKES LOTS OF PRACTICE

Information Sheet for Topic 28

Getting your healthy needs met safely, relating to yourself with compassion, and giving yourself the care you need (like using healing-focused coping skills such as grounding and separating past from present when feeling too much or too little), shifting from trauma-based thoughts to healing-focused thinking, and developing a healthy relationship with your emotions are each important parts of getting and feeling safer. Progress in each of these areas will help you get and feel safer—step by step. You'll get there—and getting there takes lots of practice.

What is a good approach to this work?

- **Go at a pace that is right for you.** When practicing, try to take what feels like a manageable next step. Remind yourself to be patient and self-compassionate. Lasting change takes practice and time! Use healthy coping skills (such as grounding) if you start feeling too much or too little.

- **If you have parts, work with them to help them understand why this is important for all of you.** Listen to and take any concerns (fears) they have seriously. Find ways to address their concerns and help make this work manageable for your parts, so that they can genuinely agree that it is OK.

- **Make early emotion-noticing and emotion-naming sessions brief** (less than a minute!) at first. You can extend the time as you get more comfortable.

Reminder: To develop healthy relationships with emotions (and parts)

Work toward relating to all parts of yourself with curiosity and compassion.

Ask yourself: What am I (my parts) feeling? Why might I (my parts) be feeling this way? Is there something I am missing? Are there things I am not paying attention to? Am I being fair? What can I do that will best help address the situation?

Remind yourself: Feelings always make sense based on what we think is happening/has happened/will happen. It is difficult to notice (and easy to minimize) things that do not fit what you are feeling. Give yourself lots of credit if you can notice something you had not before! Give yourself the care you need.

TIP: Be curious about what is best for you in the here and now, with the strengths and resources you have now as an adult. The bigger the emotion, the more important it feels, the more you want to make sure you are not missing something important before deciding what to do.

EXERCISES FOR TOPIC 28: FEELING SAFE TAKES LOTS OF PRACTICE

We hope you have been practicing using self-compassionate thoughts and behaviors and changing your responses to shame when you notice you are beginning to feel shame, are having shame-based thoughts, or are feeling a pull to follow "shame scripts." We also hope you are using your plan to keep yourself in your window of tolerance while working toward noticing feelings safely and giving yourself lots of credit for all the work you are doing to help yourself heal.

In the information sheet for Topic 28, we talked about how feeling safe takes LOTS of practice. Please review this information before continuing on.

As with all work in this program, make sure you are grounded before beginning this work, and go at a pace that is manageable for you. Check in with yourself periodically to notice your level of distress, taking breaks to ground and use healthy coping as you need to.

Are you grounded? Let's start.

Written Exercise for Topic 28: Feeling Safe Takes LOTS of Practice

Giving yourself encouragement

The process of feeling safe—including feeling safe while feeling your feelings—takes a LOT of practice. Please be gentle with yourself as you do this practice, giving yourself the care you need as you need it.

You may have spent many, many years avoiding feelings. Think about the best way to respond to a child, or a close friend, or a pet if they were learning something that was new and very difficult: You would need to give them many, many times to practice. You would want to be encouraging rather than critical. You would want to teach them that trying and practicing are important, and that it's both OK and understandable if they are not successful right away. For example, when a child learns to walk, they do not take steps right away; they begin by practicing standing still while they are holding on to a table or chair, not even moving. That may be the best way to learn how to deal with feelings: Just let yourself stand or sit still with the feelings for a little bit of time. When you are ready, you can choose to move on to the next step that feels manageable to you.

Give yourself the same gentle patience. Allow yourself to practice with little bits of feelings, gradually over time, again and again. Because you are learning something new, you may sometimes make mistakes. Try to be gentle with yourself as you commit to practicing having feelings safely to help yourself expand your window of tolerance.

Try also to help yourself remember what it means that you are now an adult: You have many more ways of coping than you did as a child, and you are now able to learn and use healthy coping skills that you could not then. There is a lot of power in being able to make healthy choices as an adult. If you choose to work to heal and get freer, and if you practice it again and again, you can make progress. You can get a healthier kind of control. Remember: One step at a time, you'll get there!

Approaching yourself like you would a child or close friend who is learning something new, please use the space below to write about how things have been going with practicing paying attention to and naming your feelings.

Allow yourself to begin by noticing and giving yourself credit for what you have done and what is working well; also see if you can notice what is helping those things work well.

_____

_____

_____

_____

_____

_____

_____

_____

While being gentle with yourself, please also write about what is still difficult, and consider which healthy skills you might use to help yourself (and your parts, if you have parts) make this process more manageable. (Doing this work often involves using all you've learned so far as part of this program. Feel free to go back to previous materials!) Again, please be gentle with yourself as you work toward your goals: Like all learning, this is a process that takes time.

_____

_____

_____

_____

_____

_____

_____

_____

_____

_____

_____

_____

_____

_____

Practice Exercise for Topic 28: Feeling Safe Takes LOTS of Practice

We encourage you to practice noticing and naming your feelings while being gentle and patient with yourself. (And remember: It does get easier with practice. Keep practicing!)

We also encourage you to continue to practice changing your responses to shame. Practice using self-compassionate thoughts and behaviors when you are beginning to feel shame, have shame-based thoughts, or feel a pull to follow shame scripts.

Give yourself credit for making progress when you are able to:

1. Notice you are feeling shame
2. Notice that trauma-based thoughts are perpetuating the shame
3. Practice self-compassionate thoughts and behaviors when you are tempted to do old shame-perpetuating behaviors (avoiding, withdrawing, or being harsh with yourself or others).

Noticing and naming feelings and replacing shaming thoughts and shame scripts with self-compassionate thoughts and behaviors takes effort and lots of practice. Give yourself credit for doing this difficult work! You can feel proud about working hard to heal.

Be patient with yourself. Lasting change takes practice and time. Keep at it!

LET THE GOOD TIMES ROLL—LEARNING HOW TO ALLOW GOOD FEELINGS AND POSITIVE EXPERIENCES

Information Sheet for Topic 29

It is difficult to truly enjoy life if you do not feel happiness, peacefulness, or pleasure at least some of the time. Doing healthy things that help you feel these feelings is an important part of getting and feeling safer.

Why might it be difficult to feel good?

- People who have experienced trauma often do not feel good before practicing healing-focused ways of helping themselves and getting healthy needs met safely.
- It is difficult to feel good feelings while (unintentionally or intentionally) suppressing feelings. When you suppress feelings, you tend to lose touch with all of your emotions, not just the ones you do not want.
- Traumatic experiences can lead people to believe that feeling good is not OK, that they don't deserve to feel good, or that having good feelings only leads to disappointment. It can seem dangerous to allow themselves to feel good. These trauma-based beliefs can lead people to not want to, or even to be afraid of, feeling good.

How can I help myself feel better?

- Help yourself shift trauma-based thoughts toward recovery-focused thinking.
- Keep practicing healing-focused ways of helping yourself when feeling too much or too little.
- Keep practicing getting your healthy needs met safely. Feeling good at least some of the time is a healthy need. **Build time into your schedule for doing healthy things that help you feel happiness, peacefulness, or pleasure at least some of the time.**
- Keep working to develop healthy relationships with all your emotions at a pace that works for you.
- Keep working to relate to yourself with healthy self-compassion.
- If you have parts, work to develop healthy relationships with all your parts. Strive to work together toward getting and feeling safer.

What are signs I might be having trauma-based thoughts?

Without minimizing things in the present that are not OK, get curious when:

- you are having an intense or overwhelming emotion
- a situation feels like or just like something from the past, or you feel you urgently need to do something
- you are having an intensely negative reaction to someone
- you are having intensely negative thoughts about yourself.

What are the most common trauma-based thoughts about feeling good?

The following beliefs are not true or fair, but they are often believed by people who have experienced trauma:

- Feeling good is not OK.
- I do not have the right to feel good.
- I do not deserve to feel good.

What are the steps to shift trauma-based thoughts to healing-focused thinking?

If you realize that you are having a trauma-based thought:

- **Give yourself credit!** It is not easy to notice that you are having a trauma-based thought.
- **Give yourself compassion and the care you need.**
- **Collect evidence** that helps you notice and remember that this trauma-based thought is not true.
- **Make a list** of any trauma-based thought(s) that you have been able to notice (even if only once!) is not true. Keep collecting evidence that helps you recognize these beliefs are not true.
- **Create recovery-focused thoughts to replace trauma-based ones, and collect evidence that the healing-focused thoughts are true.**

Each time you notice and change trauma-based thoughts, your brain gets better at noticing when you are safer. This process helps trim fear pathways in the brain and build new, calm, healthy pathways. **Each effort you make** (whether you notice or not!) **helps toward your goal.**

EXERCISES FOR TOPIC 29: LET THE GOOD TIMES ROLL—LEARNING HOW TO ALLOW GOOD FEELINGS AND POSITIVE EXPERIENCES

We hope you have been practicing being gentle and self-compassionate while paying attention to your feelings. We also hope that you have been changing your responses to shame when you notice you are beginning to feel shame, have shame-based thoughts, or feel a pull to follow shame scripts and are giving yourself lots of credit for all the work you are doing to help yourself heal.

In the information sheet for Topic 29, we talked about learning how to allow good feelings and positive experiences. Please review this information before continuing on.

As with all work in this program, make sure you are grounded before beginning this work, and go at a pace that is manageable for you. If you tend to believe that you don't deserve to feel good, that feeling good is not OK, or that having good feelings only leads to disappointment, we recommend developing a "Before, During, and After (BDA)" plan (see Topic 12, p. 97) and starting with just small amounts of emotion for very short amounts of time to prevent yourself from triggering yourself. Check in with yourself periodically to notice your level of distress, taking breaks to ground and use healthy coping as you need to.

Are you grounded? Let's start.

Written Exercise for Topic 29: Let the Good Times Roll—Learning How to Allow Good Feelings and Positive Experiences

Looking at factors that may be keeping you from feeling good

Changing beliefs is difficult, but if you allow yourself to begin to notice positive things about yourself, you can slowly begin to build a new view of yourself. Important ways to build new beliefs are to allow yourself to have positive experiences and to notice when things are OK or even good. This may be difficult if you feel like you do not have the right to feel good feelings. Or if you have not been allowing yourself to notice good things about yourself. Or if you dismiss compliments. Or if you think others don't know "the real you" if they like you. Some of you may feel like you do not deserve to get better in therapy.

If you believe any of these things, you may have ways of preventing yourself from feeling good. If you have any of these negative beliefs, we hope you will talk to your therapist about them. We encourage you to work on making small changes in your thinking. For example, if you normally say to yourself "I'm bad" or "I deserve punishment," you might shift to "I don't *always* do bad things" or "I'm trying to do things better" and remind yourself of positive things you have done.

You can also make small changes by acting slightly differently. For example, if someone compliments you, you might encourage yourself to see if there is a tiny bit of truth to what they say. Or if somebody seems to enjoy being with you, you might say to yourself, "I can notice that this person enjoys being with me this one time." Take small steps to recognize the little ways that you do things OK or even well.

Another way to nudge yourself to make changes is to notice when you say negative things to yourself. You might say to yourself, "I just judged myself." Or if you find yourself thinking, "I don't deserve to feel better," you might say, "I'm working hard to heal from trauma. It might be OK for me to feel a little bit better."

If you worry that feeling good may make you vulnerable to something bad happening, you could say, "Let me see if anything bad happens after letting myself feel a little bit better." (This is another topic that is helpful to talk to a therapist about: As we've mentioned before, we are all more likely to only notice and pay attention to things that fit with what we already believe—and this is definitely true with trauma-based beliefs. Consider re-reviewing Topics 11 and 17 with these kinds of thoughts in mind.)

People feel vulnerable when they work on changing long-held beliefs. Sometimes while trying out new ways of behaving or thinking, something stressful does happen. It does not necessarily mean that you caused the stressful thing to happen. It can feel like you are being "pushed back" for every step forward you take. Try not to be too discouraged about stressors or if your symptoms get worse after improving for a while. It is normal to have ups and downs with stress and symptoms. Gently encourage yourself to keep trying. Practice again and again. It takes a lot of practice to change habits and thinking that you have had for years.

The prompts below focus on allowing yourself to feel good feelings. As always, your safety comes first: Pay attention to your level of distress, use your plan to keep yourself in your window of tolerance (Topic 21), take breaks if you need to, and follow your healthy coping and safety plans.

Identifying and addressing factors that may be keeping you from feeling better
Some people who have experienced trauma feel uncomfortable feeling good.[1] Do you feel like you do not deserve to feel good? Or that you must criticize or punish yourself if you do feel good? Does letting yourself feel good after someone compliments you make you feel afraid or guilty? Do you worry that, if you feel good (or feel good about yourself), something bad might happen?

If you found yourself saying "yes" to any of these signs of being uncomfortable feeling pleasure, please know that each of these reactions reflects the result of believing trauma-based thoughts, which are thoughts that feel true—and may have helped you get through difficult situations you could not get away from—but are not true/no longer true/no longer helpful.

Use the space below to begin to draft more fair, healing-focused thoughts about feeling good. You may find it helpful to re-review the materials on shifting from trauma-based and shaming thoughts toward healing-focused, self-compassionate thoughts (Topics 11, 17, and 27). You may

---

[1] Informed by Lewis et al., 2004, p. 69.

also find it helpful to phrase things in a way that feels like a manageable next step, making space for feeling a little better, and then building on and revising as you feel safer doing this.

_____

_____

_____

_____

_____

_____

_____

_____

_____

_____

_____

_____

_____

Do you have a hard time believing you have the right to feel good, or does it feel dangerous to feel good?

If yes, do you find yourself doing things to prevent yourself from feeling good? What kinds of things do you notice doing to prevent yourself from feeling good?

_____

_____

_____

_____

_____

_____

Think about the kinds of things you could do instead of preventing yourself from feeling good. *(Feel free to look at the program materials.)* You can change slowly. What could you do that would be a little bit different?

_____

_____

_____

_____

_____

Some people who have experienced trauma sometimes feel so guilty about feeling better that they sabotage themselves when they start to feel better. Do you find yourself doing things that make you feel worse just when things might be getting better? What things do you find yourself doing?

_____

_____

_____

_____

_____

_____

What kinds of things could you do instead of sabotaging feeling better? What could you do that would be a little bit different?

_____

_____

_____

_____

_____

People who have experienced trauma may also forget to do safe, pleasant, and fun things that might help them feel better. What kinds of safe, pleasant, or fun things could you add to your schedule?

_____

_____

_____

_____

_____

_____

_____

Does the thought of doing things differently bring up inner conflicts? If yes, see if you can identify the concerns (fears/worries) underlying those conflicts, and write about them and ways you might address them. (Please remember to not be critical.) (This may be a good topic to discuss with your therapist.)

_____

_____

_____

_____

_____

_____

_____

_____

_____

_____

_____

_____

_____

_____

_____

For people who have parts: If you have parts, would all parts of you be willing to allow more good feelings into your life if they were absolutely sure that this could be done in a way that is safe and OK?

If not, write about why. (This may reveal more trauma-based/shaming thoughts. This may also be a good topic to discuss with your therapist.)

_____

_____

_____

_____

_____

_____

Are there any ways of doing things a bit differently (e.g., are there any pleasant activities you could add to your day or schedule) that parts could agree would be OK to try? List those here:

_____

_____

_____

_____

_____

Practice Exercise for Topic 29: Let the Good Times Roll—Learning How to Allow Good Feelings and Positive Experiences

See if you can set aside time to do some things you enjoy. Try to schedule some relaxation or free time. Try doing some of the things you listed in the written exercise. Work to not criticize yourself, or parts of yourself, when you try these activities. The goal is to give yourself permission to do them. If some of this feels like too much change too fast, see what you can do that is a little bit different.

As you go through this work, please see if you can:

- **Notice things that are OK or good, things that you do well, and ways that you are good or OK.** You may find it helpful to write down examples of these kinds of things. (If you have parts, you can also notice things that are good or OK about them.)
- **Notice when you say negative things to yourself.** You might say to yourself, "I just judged myself."
- **Make small changes in your thinking.** For example, if you normally say to yourself "I'm bad" or "I deserve punishment," you might shift to "I'm not always bad" or "I'm trying to do things better."
- **Make small changes by acting slightly differently.** For example, if someone compliments you, you might see if there is a bit of truth to what they said. Or, if somebody gives you a compliment, you might say to yourself, "It is OK to let myself feel a little bit good about what this person said."

Remember: Lasting change takes practice and time. Be patient and compassionate with yourself. Please be aware of your level of distress, and keep practicing using healthy coping and giving yourself the care you need when you need it.

Give yourself credit each time you do something toward healing. You are getting there, one step at a time! Keep at it!

Reference for Topic 29

Lewis, L., Kelly, K., & Allen, J. (2004). *Restoring hope and trust: An illustrated guide to mastering trauma.* Sidran Institute Press.

YOU HAVE LEARNED A LOT—HOW YOU CAN KEEP HEALING

Information Sheet for Topic 30

You have learned a lot over the course of this program! We hope this information has helped you and that you have begun to notice improvements in getting and feeling safer. To keep healing from the impact of trauma and to keep getting and feeling safer, please keep using the information in this program.

What have we talked about as part of this program?

- **Healthy ways to help yourself when having trauma-related reactions, symptoms, and feeling too much or too little,** including grounding; separating past from present; imagery techniques to help separate past from present and contain intrusions from the past; deep breathing; and imagery to increase a sense of peace, to notice signs of increasing distress, and to dial down overwhelming feelings.

- **The importance of self-compassion in getting and feeling safer,** and how to help yourself be more self-compassionate by giving yourself the care you need.

- **The importance of getting your healthy needs met safely,** and how to help yourself make progress toward this.

- **How to recognize and manage situations that might lead to risky, unhealthy, and unsafe behaviors—and how to break cycles of unhealthy behavior.**

- **How to manage trauma-based thoughts and crisis-level feelings.**

- **How to understand and reduce trauma-related reactions.**

- **How to shift trauma-based beliefs to healing-focused thinking.**

- **How to calm your alarm system.**

- **How to recognize and heal your window of tolerance.**

- **Reasons why feelings may be challenging, and how to help your feelings help you.**

- **How to develop healthy relationships with all of your emotions (and parts, if you have parts).**

- **How to practice having feelings safely, including how to work on shame and feeling good.**

- **How important it is to keep practicing.** Keep practicing! Each time you practice helps your brain get better at noticing when you are safer; trim fear pathways; and build new, calm, healthy pathways. Every effort you make (whether you notice or not!) helps toward your goal. Step by step, you'll get there!

EXERCISES FOR TOPIC 30: YOU HAVE LEARNED A LOT—HOW YOU CAN KEEP HEALING

We hope you have been setting aside time to do some things you enjoy and making small changes to begin to allow yourself to have some positive experiences. We also hope you have been practicing being gentle and self-compassionate while paying attention to your feelings and changing your responses to shame. Give yourself lots of credit for all the work you are doing to help yourself heal!

In the information sheet for Topic 30, we emphasized that you have learned a lot—and talked about how to keep healing. Please review this information before continuing. As with all work in this program, make sure you are grounded before beginning this work, and go at a pace that is manageable for you. Check in with yourself periodically to notice your level of distress, taking breaks to ground and use healthy coping as you need to.

Are you grounded? Let's start.

Written Exercises for Topic 30: You Have Learned a Lot—How You Can Keep Healing

You have done something important for yourself by doing the work involved in this program. We hope that you are able to ground yourself in the present moment more easily. We hope you are keeping yourself safer and are using healthy coping to deal with feelings. We also hope that you are feeling a greater sense of competence and self-compassion. One of our biggest wishes for you is that you take good care of yourself—getting your healthy needs met safely and giving yourself the care you need—by using what you have learned in this program.

We encourage you to:

- Recognize the changes you have made, and keep practicing what you have been learning to keep things going well.
- Be compassionate with yourself about any feelings you have about this part of the work ending. All your feelings are OK, even if they are mixed (meaning that some people may feel a combination of sad, happy, disappointed, or other feelings). People often have a sense of accomplishment when they finish something important—and can also feel somewhat sad or disappointed at the same time. These kinds of reactions are very understandable.
- Be compassionate with yourself if you are not yet where you'd like to be in your healing, or if you sometimes feel angry about having to keep working toward healing. This is understandable—making these kinds of changes takes lots of practice and hard work.

If you are not yet where you would like to be in your healing, that's OK! Keep practicing— you will get there! Keep nudging yourself to think about your healing as a journey. Remember that getting good at using skills that support your healing can be slow, but it does happen if you work at it!

The prompts below will help you reflect on:

- your work in this program and
- how to continue building on the progress you've made.

Written exercise 1: Reflecting on the process
What information have you learned that you have found helpful? How has it helped you?

_____

_____

_____

_____

_____

_____

_____

_____

_____

_____

Which skills have you learned that you have found helpful? How have they helped you?

_____

_____

_____

_____

_____

_____

_____

_____

_____

_____

_____

_____

_____

_____

_____

_____

What changes have you noticed as a result of practicing what you have learned?

_____

_____

_____

_____

_____

Which skills are you currently practicing most regularly?

_____

_____

_____

_____

_____

_____

_____

Written exercise 2: Developing a plan to keep building on the progress you've made
In the first exercise, you reflected on the information and skills you learned as part of this program, the impact of putting this learning into practice, and what you are currently practicing. This next exercise will help you develop a plan for continuing this important work so you can continue to build on the progress you've been making.

Review the "Overview of Topics Covered in the Program" on page 18.
Which skills would you like to practice more/might be helpful to practice more?

_____

_____

_____

_____

_____

_____

Which topics (information sheets, exercises) would you like to go back to and review?

_____

_____

_____

_____

_____

_____

What have you learned about yourself (including your parts, if you have parts) that has helped your healing?

_____

_____

_____

_____

_____

_____

What is it like to look back on all the work you have done over the course of the program? How does it feel to notice the changes you have made as a result of this information and these skills?

_____

_____

_____

_____

_____

_____

_____

How can you be compassionate with yourself about areas that you still need to work on?

_____

_____

_____

_____

_____

_____

_____

What will you do to help yourself keep the information you have been learning in mind in the future?

_____

_____

_____

_____

_____

_____

_____

_____

How will you help yourself keep practicing the skills you have been learning?

_____

_____

_____

_____

_____

_____

_____

_____

_____

_____

_____

_____

_____

_____

_____

_____

Practice Exercise for Topic 30: You Have Learned a Lot—How You Can Keep Healing

Think about all that you have learned and the hard work you have done! You have taken some very important steps for yourself. Please give yourself credit for all you have done to work on your healing.

We hope you will continue practicing these skills and working on your healing.

We encourage you to take some time to think about signs of growth that you have shown over the course of this program. Recognizing signs of growth is a very important way to help yourself stay motivated: When you recognize what you are doing right, it gives you the energy to keep working at your healing.

We also encourage you to do the things that will help you keep building on your progress. We want you to know that it matters to us that you heal. It matters to us that you keep taking care of yourself and keep working on getting healthier and getting and feeling safer.

You have begun an important process. Please keep up this good work!

We worked hard to develop this program. We wanted to help people who have experienced trauma better understand themselves and their struggles and to learn to give themselves the care and compassion they deserve. We sincerely hope it has been helpful to you. We wish you well in your continued healing.

Step by step, you are getting there!

Congratulations on completing the final module!

Thank you for continuing to make use of the program, especially during those times it was really hard to do and those times where you thought you might quit but decided not to after all. We hope this program has helped you find new ways to give yourself the care you need and deserve and that it will continue to be helpful to you as you continue on your path of healing and recovery.

We are always interested in feedback about things that helped (so we know what to keep doing) and also (and especially!) things that were confusing or things we could add or do differently to make this program more helpful. To share your feedback, please email us at feedback@ findingsolidground.net—and please keep taking good healthy care of all of who you are! (Please note that although we won't be able to respond beyond a note of appreciation for your feedback, we will be taking all feedback into consideration for future versions of this program.)

As you continue on:

Please strive to integrate what you've been learning into your daily routines. We recognize that this is much easier said than done, so please be patient with yourself as you work toward getting better and better at:

- getting your healthy needs met safely
- noticing where you are in your window of tolerance and recognizing early warning signs
- treating yourself with compassion and giving yourself the care you need, including using healthy coping (such as grounding and separating past from present) to manage difficult situations, break the cycle of unhealthy behavior, reduce trauma-related reactions, and heal trauma's impact on the brain
- recognizing and addressing trauma-based thoughts
- improving your relationship with your emotions and all of who you are
- recognizing shaming thoughts and shame-driven behaviors and replacing them with self-compassionate thoughts and behaviors
- increasing positive experiences
- noticing and giving yourself credit for progress.

Step by step, you're getting there!

RESOURCES

RECOVERING AND HEALING FROM TRAUMA AND THE PRINCIPLES OF TRAUMA-INFORMED CARE

What are the stages involved in healing and recovering from trauma?

1. **Symptom Management and Stabilization** *Learning healthy, healing-focused ways to manage trauma-related reactions and symptoms—the focus of this program.*

2. **Processing the Impact of Trauma** *Only manageable with the benefit of consistently being able to use healthy, healing-focused ways to manage trauma-related reactions and symptoms.*

3. **Reconnection** *Reconnecting with yourself and others with increased self-understanding and compassion after processing.*

What are the principles of trauma-informed care?

- **Safety** (physical and emotional)
- **Trustworthiness** (including transparency about what you are doing and why)
- **Collaboration** (through curiosity and mutuality)
- **Empowerment** (through encouraging voice and choice)
- **Attentiveness to Cultural, Historical, and Gender-Related Issues** (i.e., trauma; including racism, sexism, LGBTQIA discrimination)
- **Peer Support and Mutual Self-Help** (learning and working together)

EXTERNAL RESOURCES

Urgent Help Resources

- National Suicide Prevention Lifeline: *1-800-273-TALK (8255)*
- National Domestic Violence Hotline: *thehotline.org*
- National Sexual Assault Hotline: *www.rainn.org/get-help*

Therapist-Finding Resources

- International Society for the Study of Trauma and Dissociation's Find-A-Therapist Resource: *isstd.connectedcommunity.org/network/network-find-a-professional*
- International Society for Traumatic Stress Studies' Clinician Directory: *istss.org/public-resources/find-a-clinician.aspx*

Online Resources for Survivors of Trauma

- Adult Survivors of Child Abuse: *www.ascasupport.org*
- Trauma support resources from David Baldwin's Trauma Information Pages: *www.trauma-pages.com/support.php*
- Male Survivors: Overcoming Sexual Victimization of Boys and Men: *www.malesurvivor.org*
- 1in6 (for men who have been sexually abused or assaulted): *1in6.org*
- National Center for PTSD: *www.ptsd.va.gov*
- Sidran Institute: Traumatic Stress Education and Advocacy: *www.sidran.org*
- Survivors Network of Those Abused by Priests: *www.snapnetwork.org*

Online Resources for Information About Trauma and Dissociation

- *www.teachtrauma.com*: Facts about psychological trauma, including types of trauma, dissociation, traumatic memory, debates in the trauma field; slideshows for educators; evaluations of textbooks' coverage of trauma; classroom activities to teach about trauma; and additional resources
- International Society for the Study of Trauma and Dissociation: *www.isst-d.org*
- International Society for Traumatic Stress Studies: *www.istss.org*
- American Psychological Association Trauma Division (Division 56): *www.apatraumadivision.org*
- European Society for Trauma & Dissociation: *www.estd.org*
- National Child Traumatic Stress Network: *www.nctsn.org*
- Blue Knot Foundation in Australia: *www.blueknot.org.au*

BOOKS ON COPING WITH AND RECOVERING FROM TRAUMA

Allen, J. G. (2005). *Coping with trauma: Hope through understanding* (2nd ed.). American Psychiatric Publishing, Inc.

Bass, E., & Davis, L. (2012). *Beginning to heal (rev. ed.): A first book for men and women who were sexually abused as children.* HarperCollins.

Boon, S., Steele, K., & van der Hart, O. (2011). *Coping with trauma-related dissociation: Skills training for patients and therapists.* W. W. Norton & Company.

Brown, L. S. (2012). *Your turn for care: Surviving the aging and death of the adults who harmed you.* CreateSpace Independent Publishing Platform.

Brown, L. S. (2015). *Not the price of admission: Healthy relationships after childhood trauma.* CreateSpace Independent Publishing Platform.

Copeland, M. E., & M. Harris. (2000). *Healing the trauma of abuse: A women's workbook.* New Harbinger Publications, Inc.

Cori, J. K. (2008). *Healing from trauma: A survivor's guide to understanding your symptoms and reclaiming your life.* Da Capo Press.

Courtois, C. A. (2015). *It's not you, it's what happened to you.* Elements Behavioral Health.

Davis, L. (1991). *Allies in healing: When the person you love was sexually abused as a child.* HarperCollins.

Davis, L. (1991). *The courage to heal workbook: A guide for women and men survivors of child sexual abuse.* Harper Perennial.

Freyd, J. J., & Birrell, P. J. (2013). *Blind to betrayal: Why we fool ourselves—we aren't being fooled.* John Wiley & Sons Inc.

Lew, M. (2004). *Victims no longer: The classic guide for men recovering from sexual child abuse* (2nd ed.). HarperCollins.

Lewis, L., Kelly, K., & Allen, J. G. (2004). *Restoring hope and trust: An illustrated guide to mastering trauma.* Sidran Press.

Maltz, W. (2012). *The sexual healing journey: A guide for survivors of sexual abuse* (3rd ed.). HarperCollins.

Marich, J. (2020). *Trauma and the 12 steps: An inclusive guide to enhancing recovery* (revised and expanded ed.). North Atlantic Books.

Matsakis, A. (1996). *I can't get over it: A handbook for trauma survivors* (2nd ed.). New Harbinger Publications, Inc.

Matsakis, A. (1998). *Trust after trauma: A guide to relationships for survivors and those who love them.* New Harbinger Publications, Inc.

Matsakis, A. (1999). *Survivor guilt: A self-help guide.* New Harbinger Publications.

Miller, D. (2003). *Your surviving spirit: A spiritual workbook for coping with trauma.* New Harbinger Publications.

Miller, D., & L. Guidry. (2001). *Addictions and trauma recovery: Healing the body, mind & spirit.* W. W. Norton & Company.

Najavits, L. (2002). *A woman's addiction workbook: Your guide to in-depth healing.* New Harbinger Publications.

Najavits, L. (2019). *Finding your best self: Recovery from addiction, trauma, or both* (rev. ed.). Guilford Press.

Pennebaker, J. (1997). *Opening up: The healing power of expressing emotions* (2nd ed.). Guilford Press.

Pennebaker, J. W. (2004). *Writing to heal: A guided journal for recovering from trauma & emotional upheaval.* New Harbinger Publications, Inc.

Siegel, D. J. (2007). *The mindful brain: Reflection and attunement in the cultivation of well-being.* W. W. Norton & Company.

Siegel, D. J. (2010). *Mindsight: The new science of personal transformation.* Bantam.

Vermilyea, E. G. (2013). *Growing beyond survival: A self-help toolkit for managing traumatic stress.* Sidran Institute.

Williams, M. B., & Poijula, S. (2002). *The PTSD workbook: Simple, effective techniques for overcoming traumatic stress symptoms.* New Harbinger Publications.

BOOKS, CHAPTERS, AND ARTICLES ON TREATMENT OF COMPLEX TRAUMA-RELATED DISORDERS

Allen, J. G. (2013). *Restoring mentalizing in attachment relationships: Treating trauma with plain old therapy* (1st ed.). American Psychiatric Publishing, Inc.

Brand, B. L., Loewenstein, R. J., & Lanius, R. A. (2014). Treatment of dissociative identity disorder. In G. O. Gabbard (Ed.), *Gabbard's treatment of psychiatric disorders* (5th ed., pp. 439–458). American Psychiatric Press.

Briere, J. N., & Scott, C. (2015). *Principles of trauma therapy: A guide to symptoms, evaluation, and treatment* (2nd ed., DSM-5 update). Sage Publications, Inc.

Chefetz, R. A. (2015). *Intensive psychotherapy for persistent dissociative processes: The fear of feeling real.* W. W. Norton & Co.

Chu, J. A. (2011). *Rebuilding shattered lives: Treating complex PTSD and dissociative disorders* (2nd ed.). John Wiley & Sons Inc.

Cloitre, M., Cohen, L. R., Ortigo, K. M., Jackson, C., & Koenen, K. C. (2020). *Treating survivors of childhood abuse and interpersonal trauma: STAIR narrative therapy* (2nd ed.). Guilford Press.

Cloitre, M., Courtois, C. A., Charuvastra, A., Carapezza, R., Stolbach, B. C., & Green, B. L. (2011). Treatment of complex PTSD: Results of the ISTSS expert clinician survey on best practices. *Journal of Traumatic Stress, 24*(6), 615–627.

Cloitre, M., Courtois, C. A., Ford, J. D., Green, B. L., Alexander, P., Briere, J., Herman, J. L., Lanius, R., Stolbach, B. C., Spinazzola, J., Van der Kolk, B. A., & Van der Hart, O. (2012). *The ISTSS Expert Consensus Treatment Guidelines for Complex PTSD in Adults.* https://istss.org/ISTSS_Main/media/Documents/ComplexPTSD.pdf

Courtois, C. A. (2010). *Healing the incest wound: Adult survivors in therapy (rev. ed.)*. W. W. Norton.

Courtois, C. A., & Ford, J. D. (2009). *Treating complex traumatic stress disorders: An evidence-based guide*. Guilford Press.

Courtois, C. A., & Ford, J. D. (2013). *Treatment of complex trauma: A sequenced, relationship-based approach*. Guilford Press.

Daitch, C. (2007). *Affect regulation toolbox: Practical and effective hypnotic interventions for the over-reactive client*. W. W. Norton & Co.

Fisher, J. (2017). *Healing the fragmented selves of trauma survivors: Overcoming internal self-alienation*. Routledge.

Ford, J. D., & Courtois, C. A. (Eds.). (2020). *Treating complex traumatic stress disorders: Scientific foundations and therapeutic models* (2nd ed.). Guilford Press.

Forner, C. C. (2017). *Dissociation, mindfulness, and creative meditations: Trauma-informed practices to facilitate growth*. Routledge/Taylor & Francis Group.

Frewen, P. A., & Lanius, R. (2015). *Healing the traumatized self: Consciousness, neuroscience, treatment*. W. W. Norton & Co.

Freyd, J. J. (1996). *Betrayal trauma: The logic of forgetting childhood abuse*. Harvard.

Gartner, R. B. (2018). *Understanding the sexual betrayal of boys and men: The trauma of sexual abuse*. Routledge.

Gartner, R. B. (2018). *Healing sexually betrayed men and boys: Treatment for sexual abuse, assault, and trauma*. Routledge.

Gold, S. N. (2000). *Not trauma alone: Therapy for child abuse survivors in family and social context*. Brunner-Routledge.

Gold, S. N. (2020). *Contextual trauma therapy: Overcoming traumatization and reaching full potential*. American Psychological Association.

Harris, M. (1998). *Trauma recovery and empowerment: A clinician's guide for working with women in groups*. Free Press.

Herman, J. L. (2015). *Trauma and recovery: The aftermath of violence—from domestic abuse to political terror*. Basic Books.

Howell, E. F. (2005). *The dissociative mind*. Analytic Press/Taylor & Francis Group.

Howell, E. F. (2011). *Understanding and treating dissociative identity disorder: A relational approach*. Routledge/Taylor & Francis Group.

International Society for the Study of Trauma and Dissociation (ISSTD). (2011). Guidelines for treating dissociative identity disorder in adults, third revision. *Journal of Trauma and Dissociation, 12*(2), 115–187. doi:10.1080/15299732.2011.537247

Kezelman, C., & Stavropoulos, P. (2019). *Practice guidelines for treatment of complex trauma and trauma informed care and service delivery*. Blue Knot Foundation (ASCA). www.blueknot.org.au

Kinsler, P. J. (2018). *Complex psychological trauma: The centrality of the relationship*. Routledge.

Kluft, R. P., & Fine, C. G. (1993). *Clinical perspectives on multiple personality disorder*. American Psychiatric Press.

Lanius, U. F., Paulsen, S. L., & Corrigan, F. M. (2014). *Neurobiology and treatment of traumatic dissociation: Toward an embodied self.* Springer Publishing Company.

Levine, P. A., & Frederick, A. (1997). *Waking the tiger: Healing trauma.* North Atlantic Books.

Linehan, M. M. (2015). *DBT® skills training manual* (2nd ed.). Guilford Press.

Linehan, M. M. (2015). *DBT® skills training handouts and worksheets* (2nd ed.). Guilford Press.

Loewenstein, R. J. (2006). DID 101: A hands-on clinical guide to the stabilization phase of dissociative identity disorder treatment. *Psychiatric Clinics of North America, 29*(1), 305–332.

Loewenstein, R. J. (2014). Dissociative amnesia. In G. O. Gabbard (Ed.), *Gabbard's treatments of psychiatric disorders* (pp. 471–478). American Psychiatric Publishing, Inc.

Loewenstein, R. J., Frewen, P. A., & Lewis-Fernández, R. (2017). Dissociative disorders. In B. J. Sadock, V. A. Sadock, & P. Ruiz (Eds.), *Kaplan & Sadock's comprehensive textbook of psychiatry* (10th ed., Vol. 1, pp. 1866–1952). Wolters Kluwer/Lippincott Williams & Wilkins.

Mosquera, D. (2019). *Working with voices and dissociative parts: A trauma-informed approach.* Institute for the Treatment of Trauma and Personality Disorders. www.intra-tp.com

Najavits, L. M. (2002). *Seeking safety: A treatment manual for PTSD and substance abuse.* Guilford Press.

Ogden, P., & Fisher, J. (2015). *Sensorimotor psychotherapy: Interventions for trauma and attachment.* W. W. Norton & Co.

Ogden, P., Minton, K., & Pain, C. (2006). *Trauma and the body: A sensorimotor approach to psychotherapy.* W. W. Norton & Company.

Putnam, F. W. (1989). *Diagnosis and treatment of multiple personality disorder.* Guilford.

Putnam, F. W. (1997). *Dissociation in children and adolescents: A developmental model.* Guilford.

Putnam, F. W. (2016). *The way we are: How states of mind influence our identities, personality, and potential for change.* International Psychoanalytic Books.

Rothschild, B. (2000). *The body remembers: The psychophysiology of trauma and trauma treatment.* W. W. Norton & Company.

Rothschild, B. (2017). *The body remembers: Revolutionizing trauma treatment* (Vol. 2). W. W. Norton & Co.

Schore, A. N. (2003). *Affect dysregulation and disorders of the self.* W. W. Norton & Company.

Schwarz, R. (2002). *Tools for transforming trauma.* Brunner-Routledge.

Siegel, D. J. (2015). *The developing mind* (3rd ed.): *How relationships and the brain interact to shape who we are.* Guilford Press.

Silberg, J. L. (2013). *The child survivor: Healing developmental trauma and dissociation.* Routledge/Taylor & Francis Group.

Steele, K., Boon, S., & van der Hart, O. (2017). *Treating trauma-related dissociation: A practical, integrative approach.* W. W. Norton & Co.

Steinberg, M. (1994). *Interviewer's guide to the Structured Clinical Interview for DSM-IV Dissociative Disorders (SCID-D)* (rev. ed.). American Psychiatric Association.

Steinberg, M. (1995). *Handbook for the assessment of dissociation: A clinical guide.* American Psychiatric Press.

Steinberg, M. (2000). *The stranger in the mirror: Dissociation—the hidden epidemic.* Cliff Street/Harper-Collins.

van der Hart, O., Nijenhuis, E. R. S., & Steele, K. (2006). *The haunted self.* W. W. Norton & Co.

van der Kolk, B. A. (2014). *The body keeps the score: Brain, mind, and body in the healing of trauma.* Viking.

Walker, D., Courtois, C. A., & Aten, J. (Eds.) (2015). *Spirituality oriented psychotherapy for trauma.* American Psychological Association Press.

ABOUT THE AUTHORS

Hugo J. Schielke, Ph.D., is Trauma Services Development Lead for Homewood Health Centre and the Centre's Traumatic Stress Injury & Concurrent Program in Guelph, Ontario. He specializes in the assessment and treatment of trauma-related disorders, and his work is informed by his post-doctoral fellowship at The Trauma Disorders Program at Sheppard Pratt Health System and his involvement with the California Department of State Hospitals' Trauma-Informed Care Project. His research is focused on the treatment of trauma-related disorders, psychotherapy process, and the relational components of psychotherapy.

Bethany L. Brand, Ph.D., a professor at Towson University, is an expert in trauma disorders and dissociation. She serves on international and national task forces developing guidelines for the assessment and treatment of trauma disorders. Dr. Brand's research focuses on a series of international dissociative disorders treatment studies (TOP DD studies), assessment methods for distinguishing dissociative disorders from other conditions including malingering, training therapists about treating trauma, and the assessment of the accuracy and adequacy of textbooks' coverage of trauma. In her private practice, Dr. Brand treats complex trauma patients and serves as a forensic expert in trauma-related cases.

Ruth A. Lanius, M.D., Ph.D., is a psychiatry professor and Harris-Woodman Chair at Western University of Canada, where she directs the Clinical Research Program for PTSD. Ruth has over 25 years of clinical and research experience with trauma-related disorders. Ruth has received numerous research and teaching awards, including the Banting Award for Military Health Research. She has published over 150 research articles and book chapters focusing on brain adaptations to psychological trauma and novel adjunct treatments for PTSD. Ruth has co-authored *The Effects of Early Life Trauma on Health and Disease: The Hidden Epidemic* and *Healing the Traumatized Self: Consciousness, Neuroscience, Treatment.*